DOULA
DOODLES 1

an adult colouring book for expectant mothers

doulas midwives and birth junkies

illustrated by

Jemmais Keval-Baxter

Matrilineal Ink

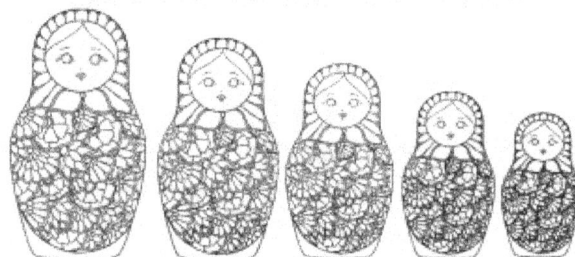

www.matrilineal.cl

ISBN 978-1-9998071-0-8

Other books by Jemmais Keval Baxter:

A Doulas Guide to Nutrition
A Doulas Guide to the Placenta
A Doulas Guide to Menstruation
A Doulas Guide to Education
A Doulas Guide to Breastfeeding

and
Ho'oponopono Birth:
Meditations on Ho'oponopono for Pregnancy and Childbirth

More information and resources can be found at
www.hooponoponodoula.com

The womb of the mother is the most sacred place on earth.

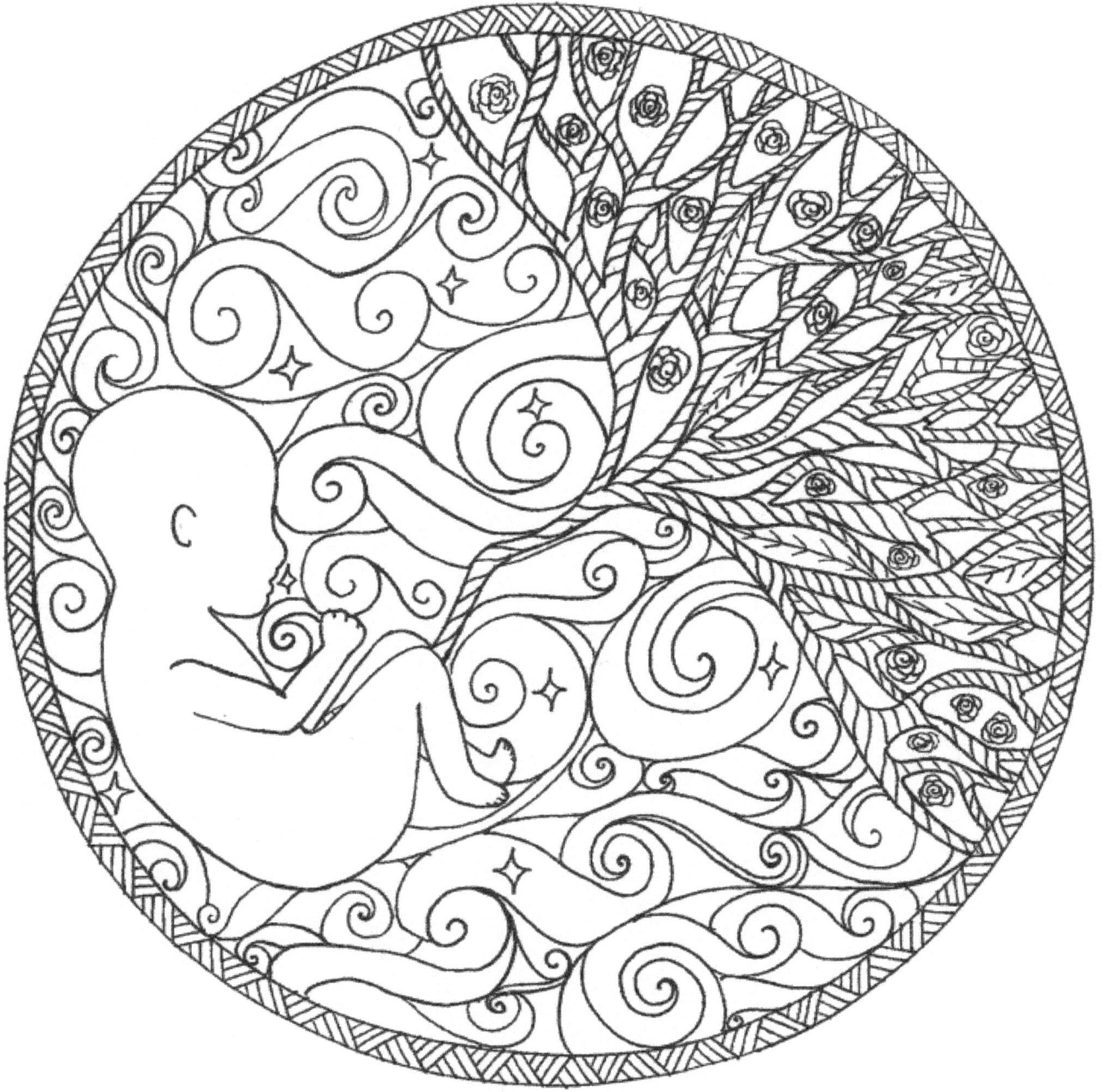

"Heaven lies at the feet of a mother."

Prophet Muhammad

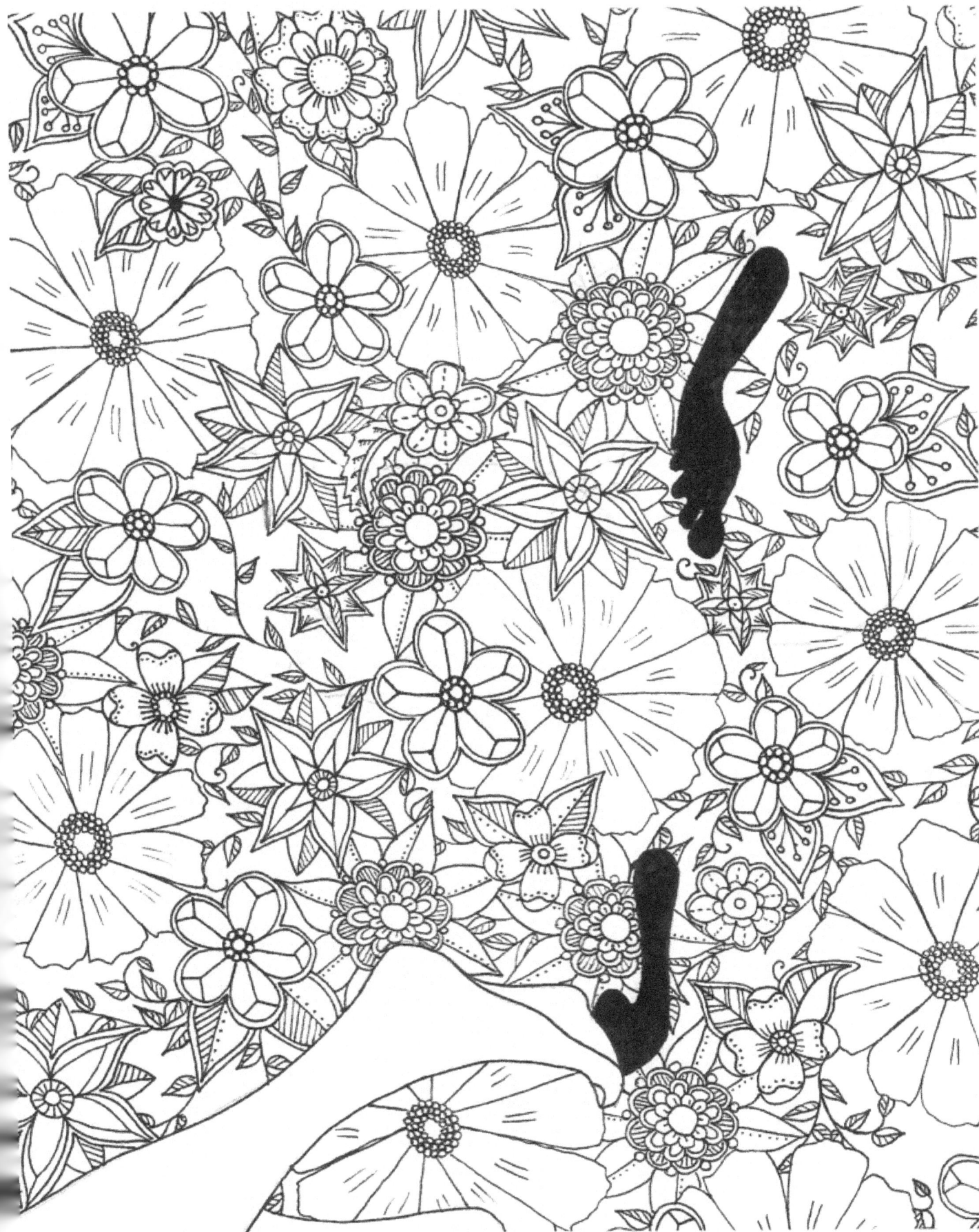

When you are a mother, you are never really alone in your thoughts. A mother always has to think twice, once for herself and once for her child.

Sophia Loren

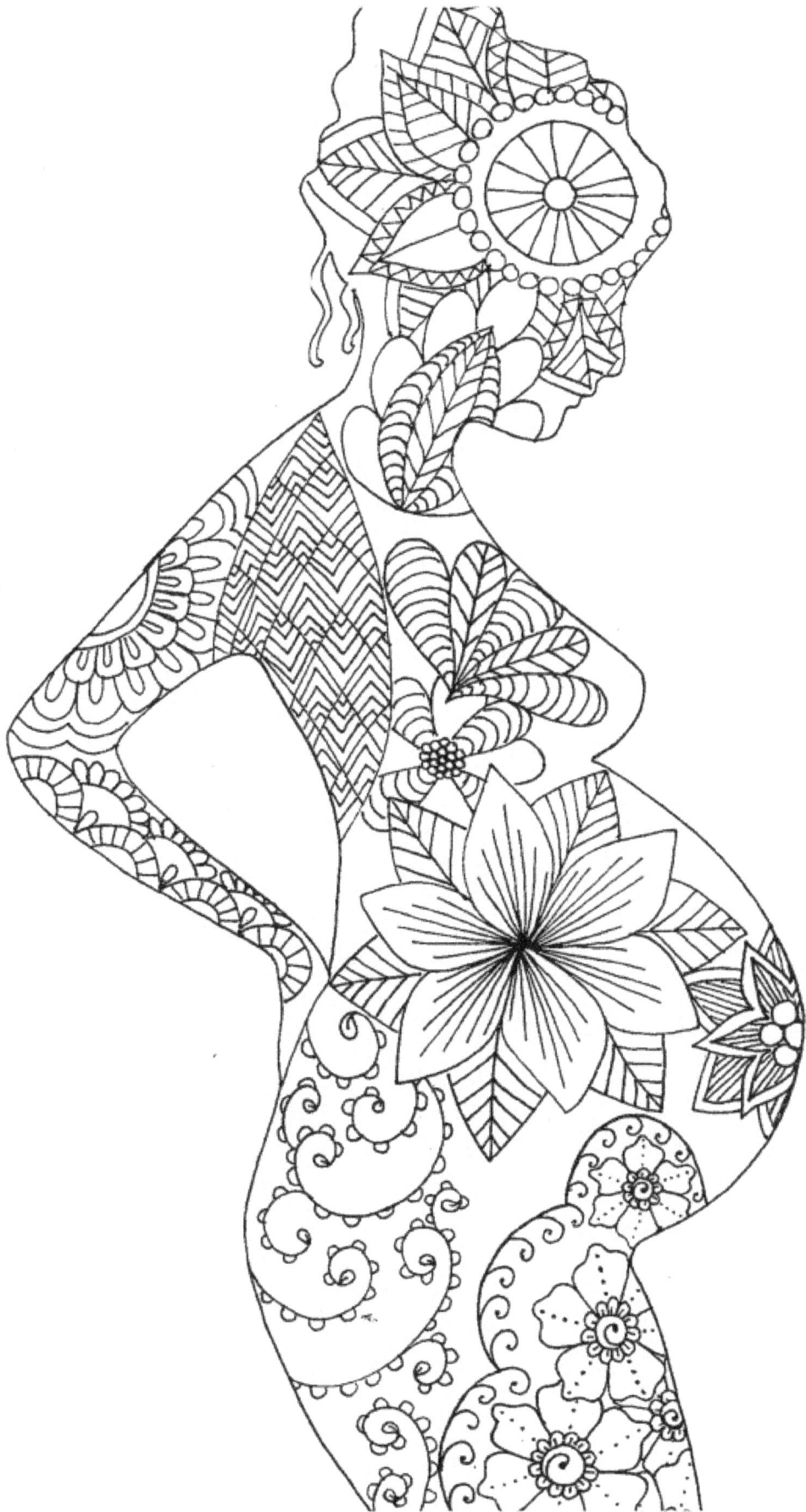

"The seeds of life inside my womb were present at my birth; a gift from mother's mother, on back to Mother Earth."

— Patricia Robin Woodruff

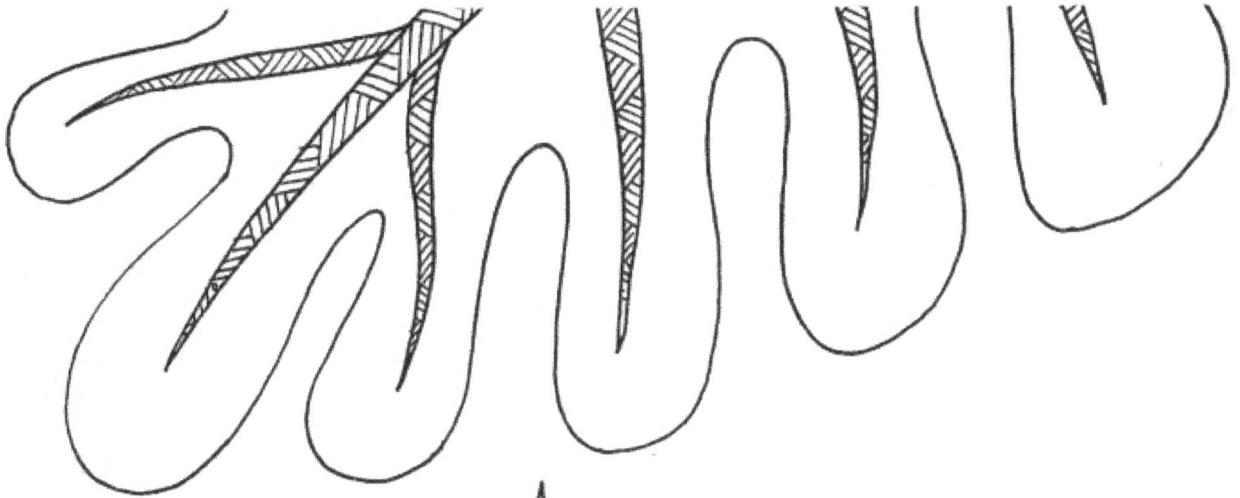

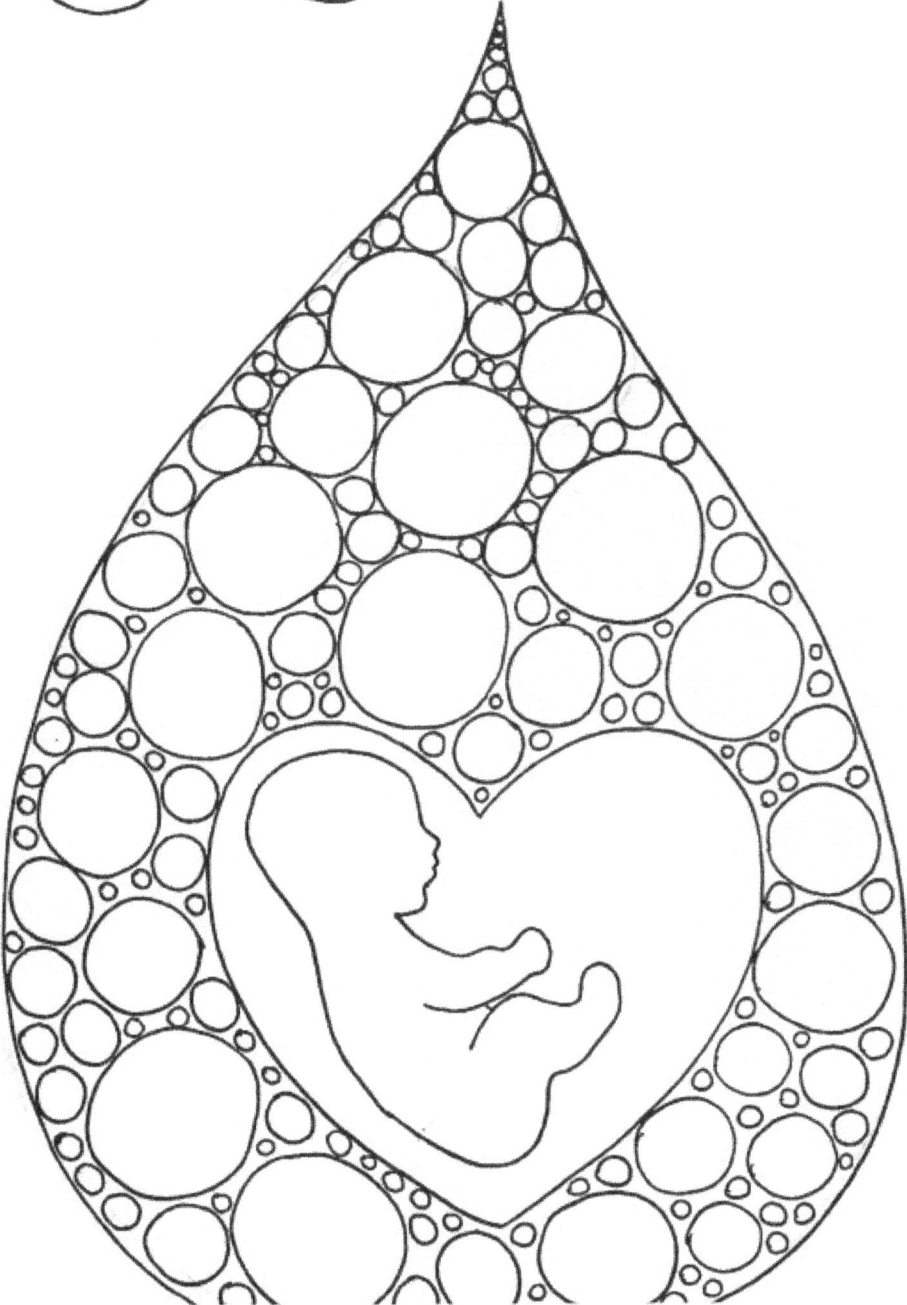

"Giving birth and being born brings us into the essence of creation, where the human spirit is courageous and bold and the body, a miracle of wisdom."

– Harriette Hartigan

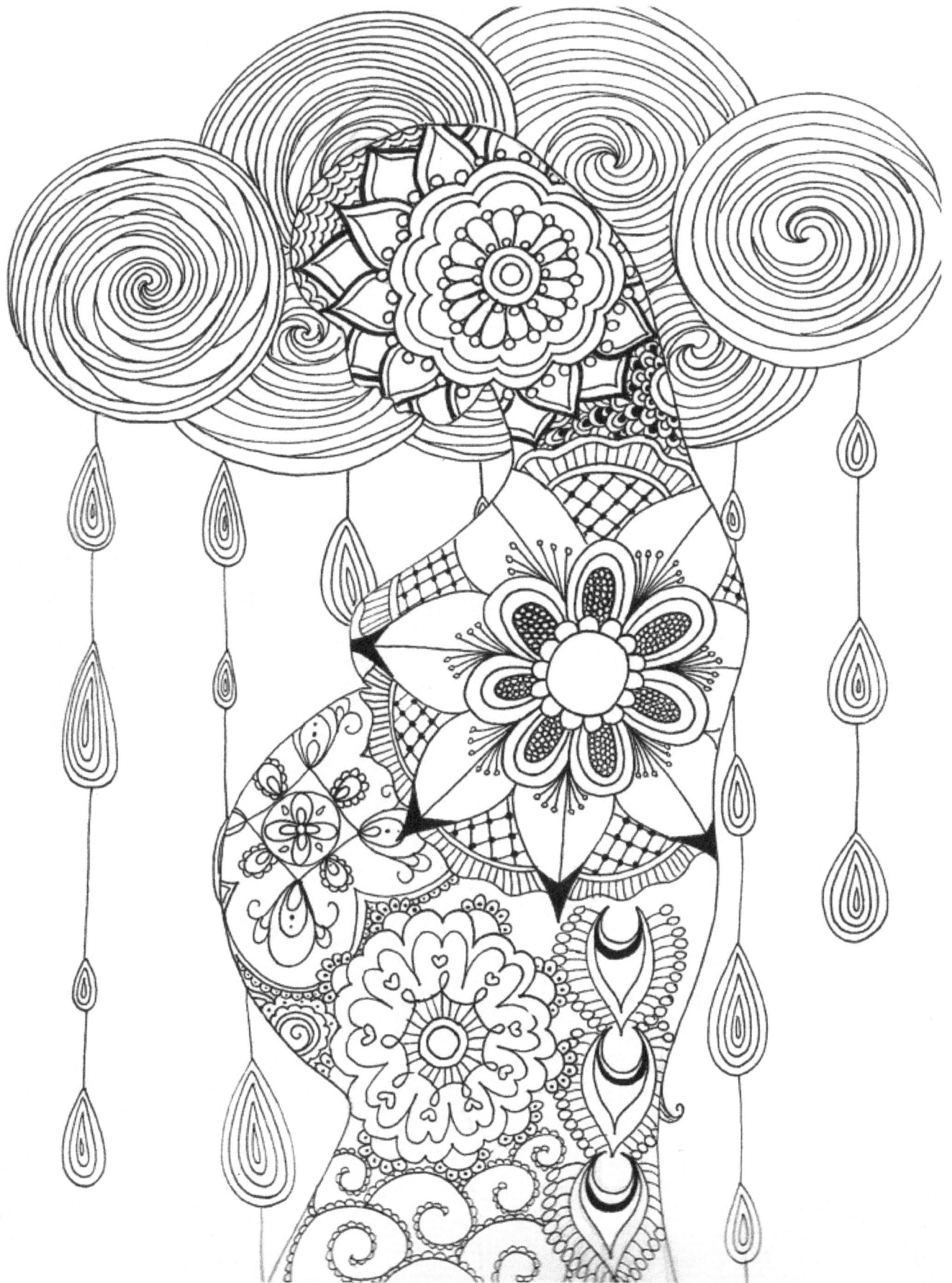

"All the time we wondered and wondered, who is this person coming, growing, turning, floating, swimming deep, deep inside?"

– Crescent Dragonwagon

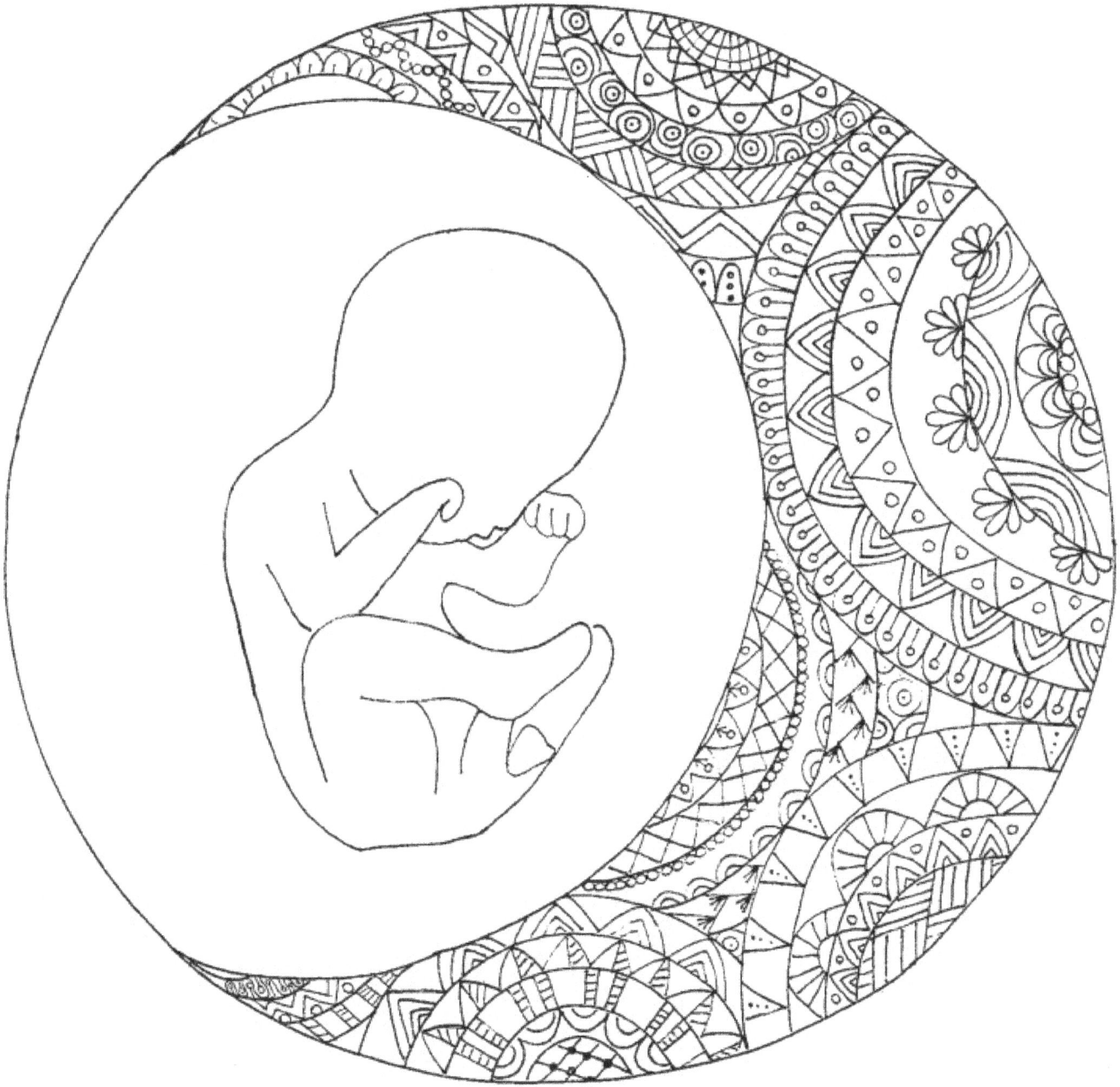

"To be pregnant is to be vitally alive, thoroughly woman, and distressingly inhabited. Soul and spirit are stretched – along with body – making pregnancy a time of transition, growth, and profound beginnings."

– Anne Christian Buchanan

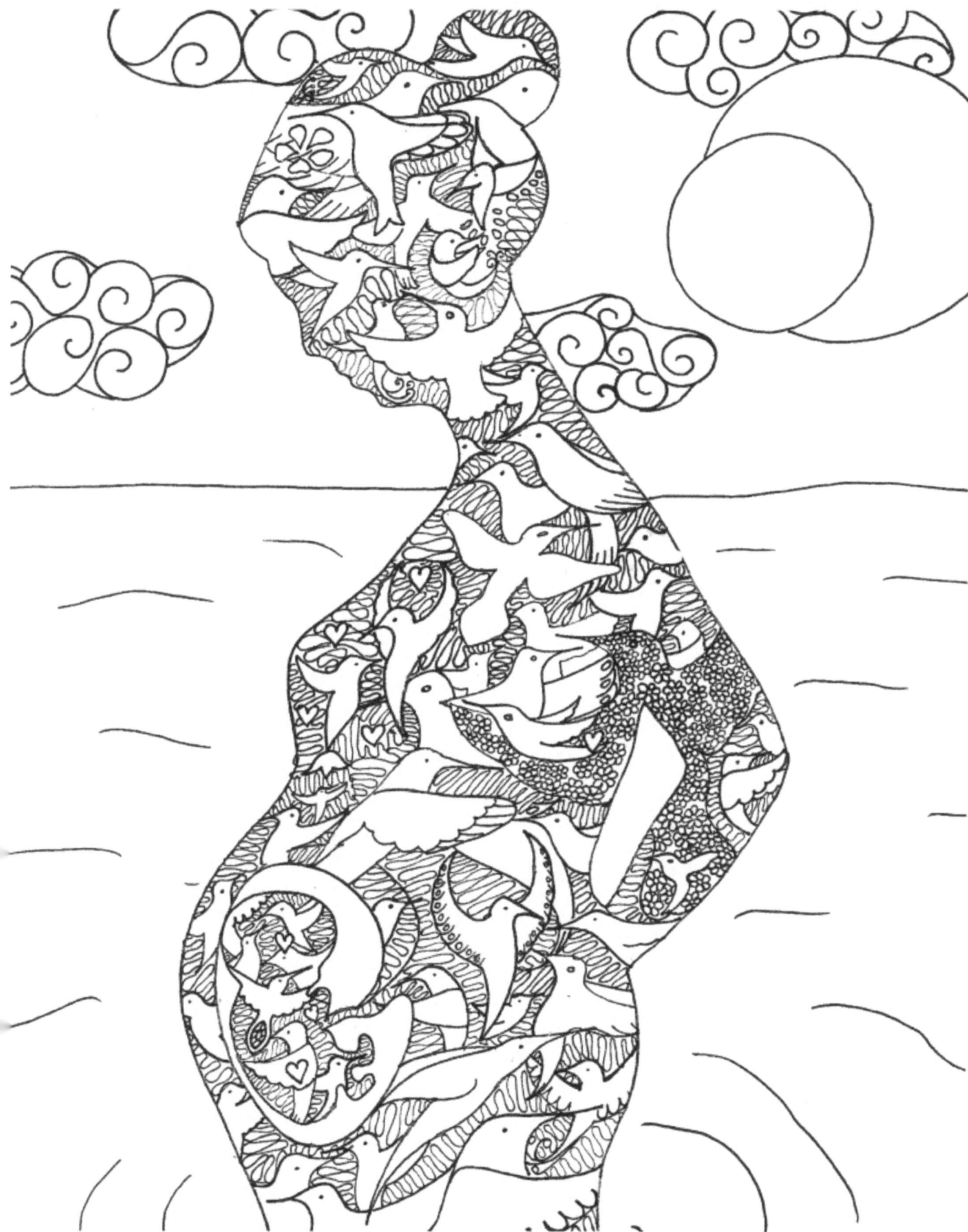

Only love is all maroon

…..Sky is womb and she's the moon"

Bon Iver

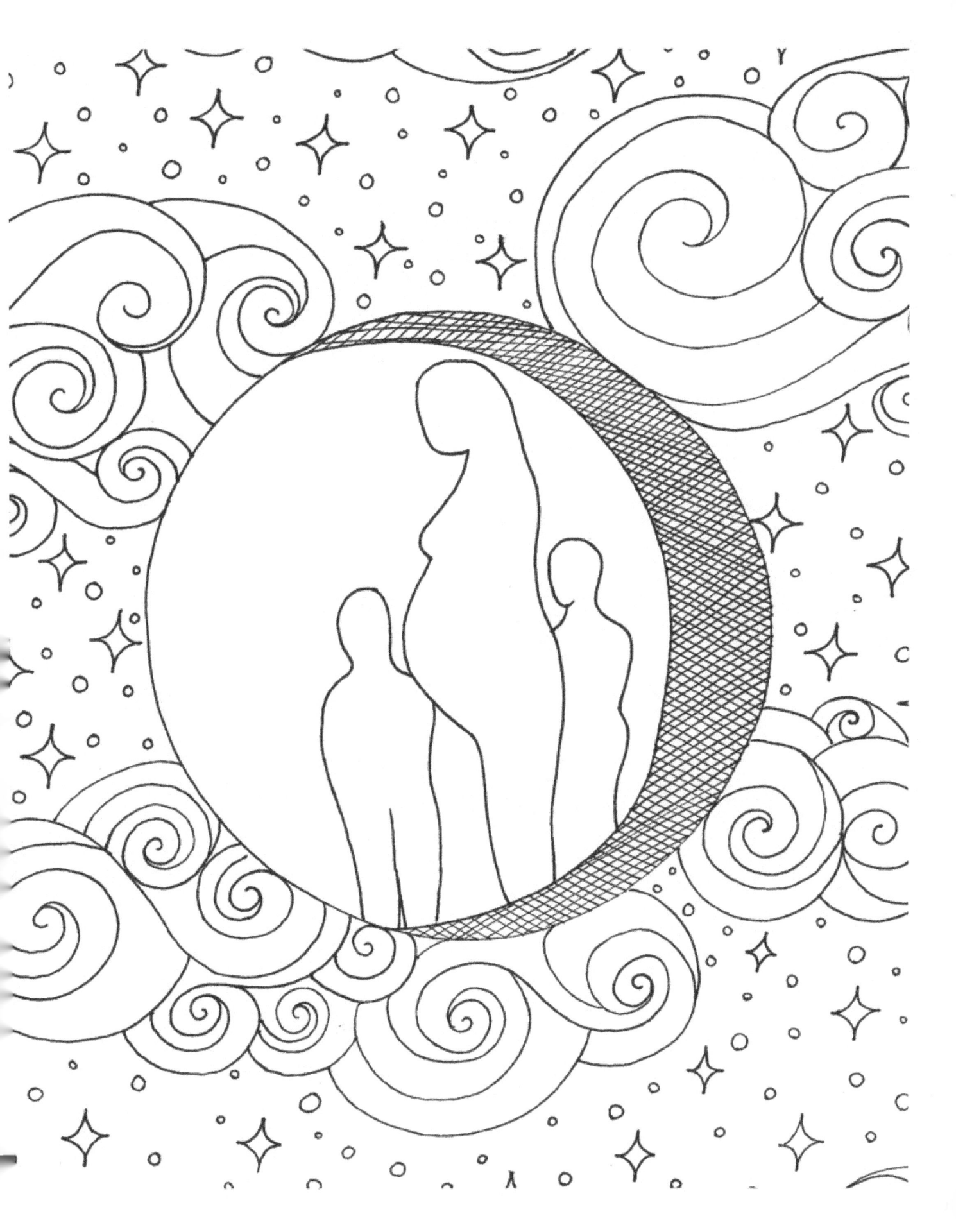

A grand adventure is about to begin.

– Winnie the Pooh

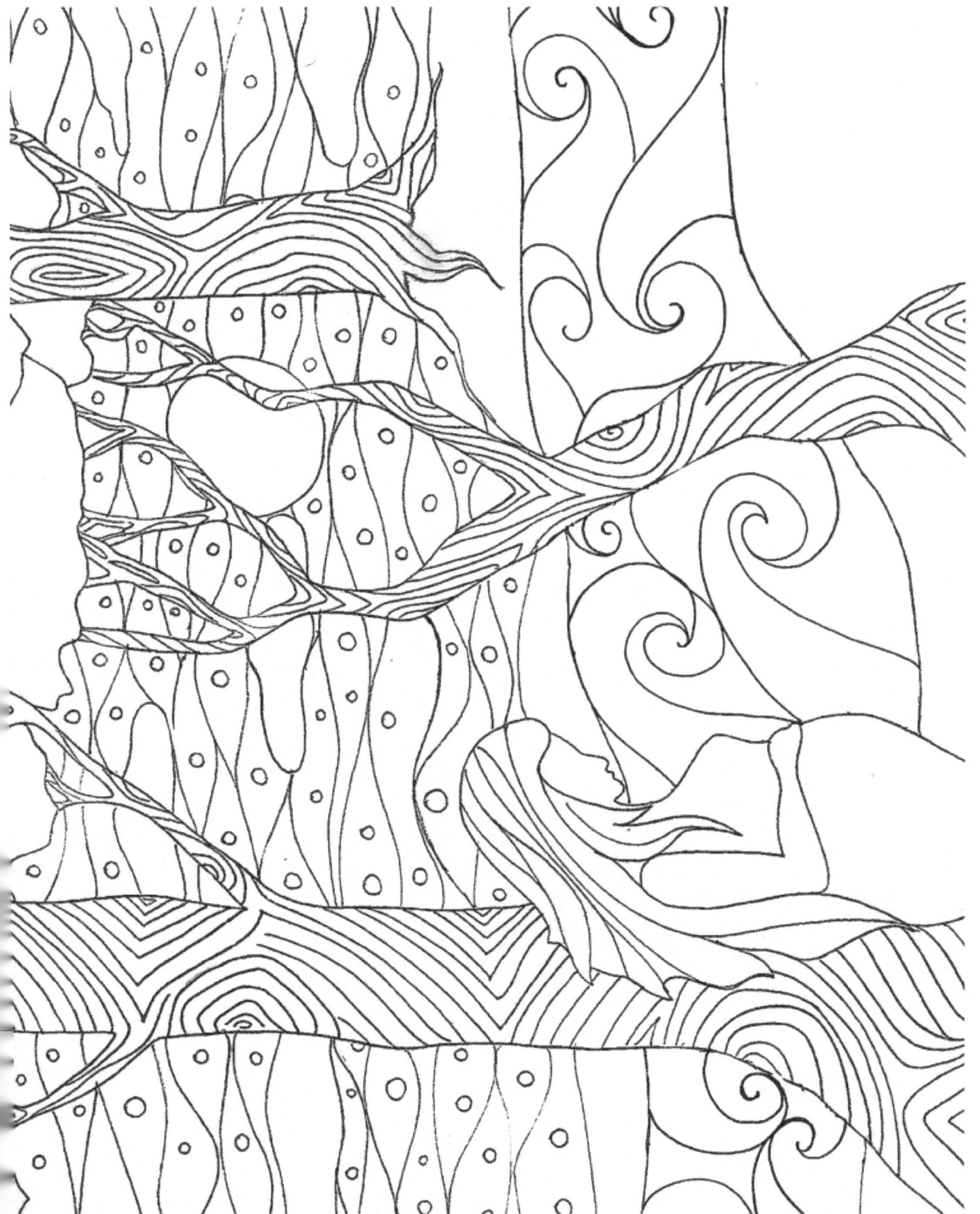

Now my belly is as noble as my heart.

Gabriela Mistral

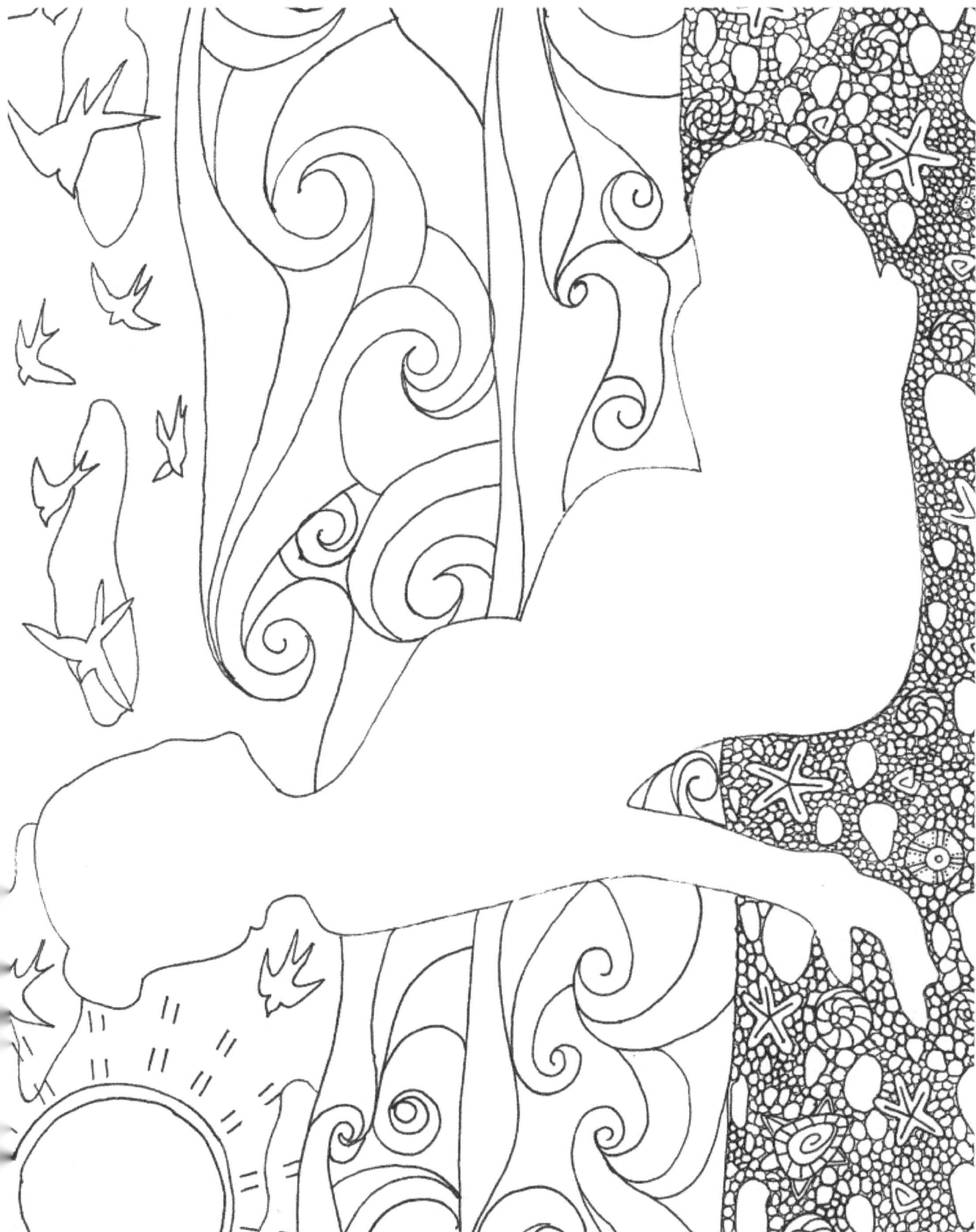

In the watery world of the unborn, the placenta beats out an ancient rhythm, tethering us to life itself.

Amy stenzel

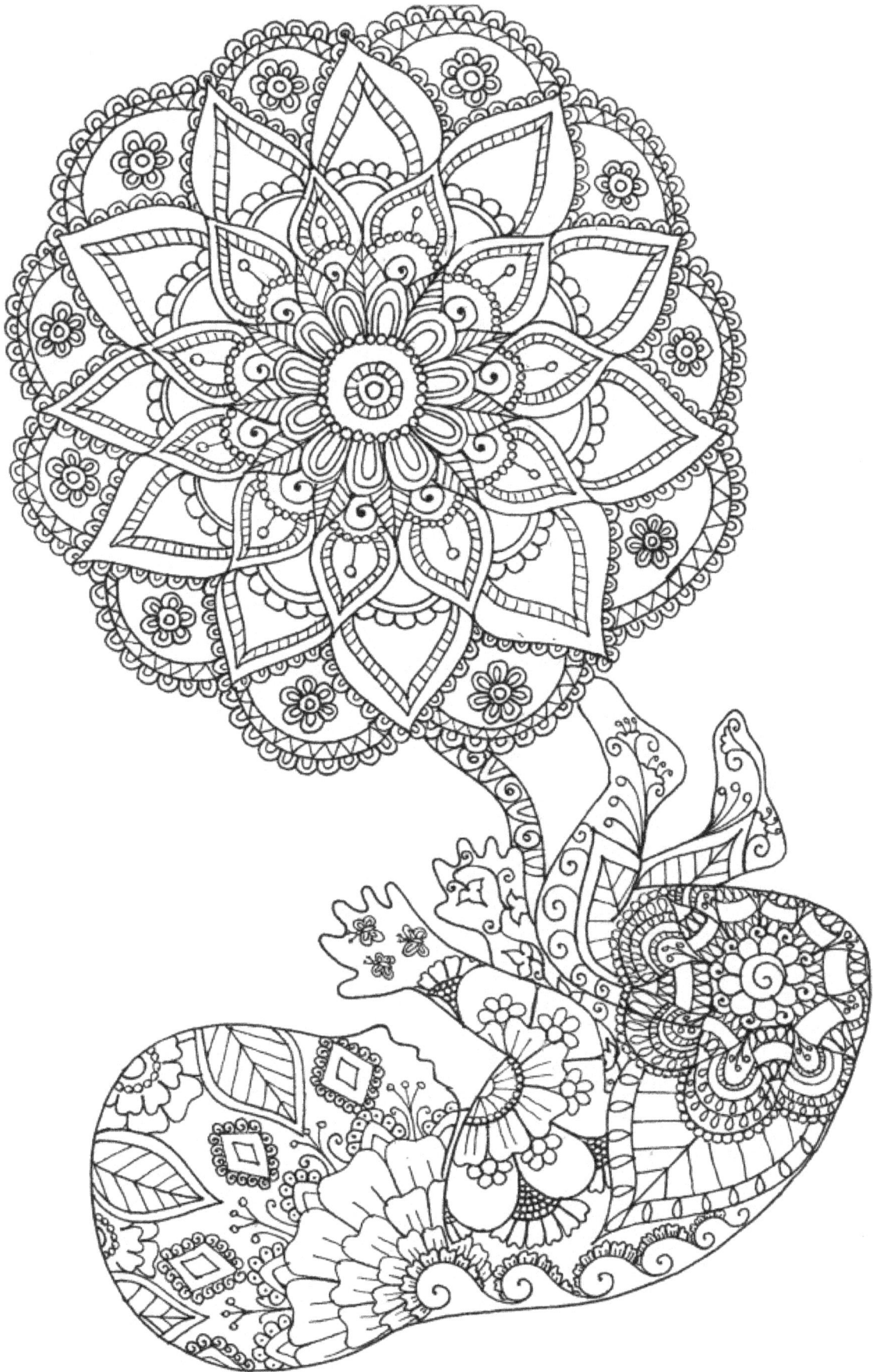

Motherhood: All love begins and ends there.

Robert Browning

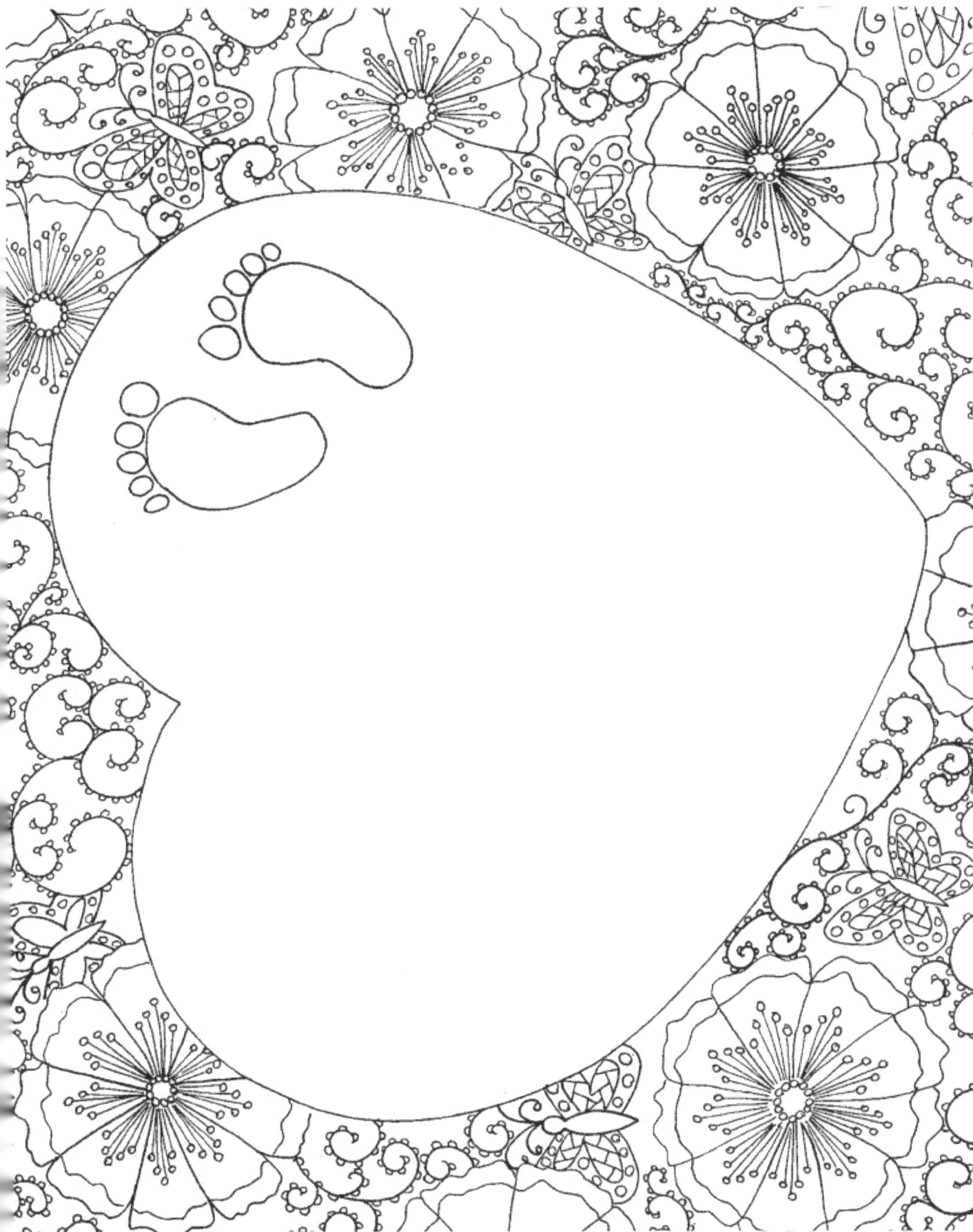

There is nothing like a newborn baby to renew your spirit and to buttress your resolve to make the world a better place.

Virginia Kelley

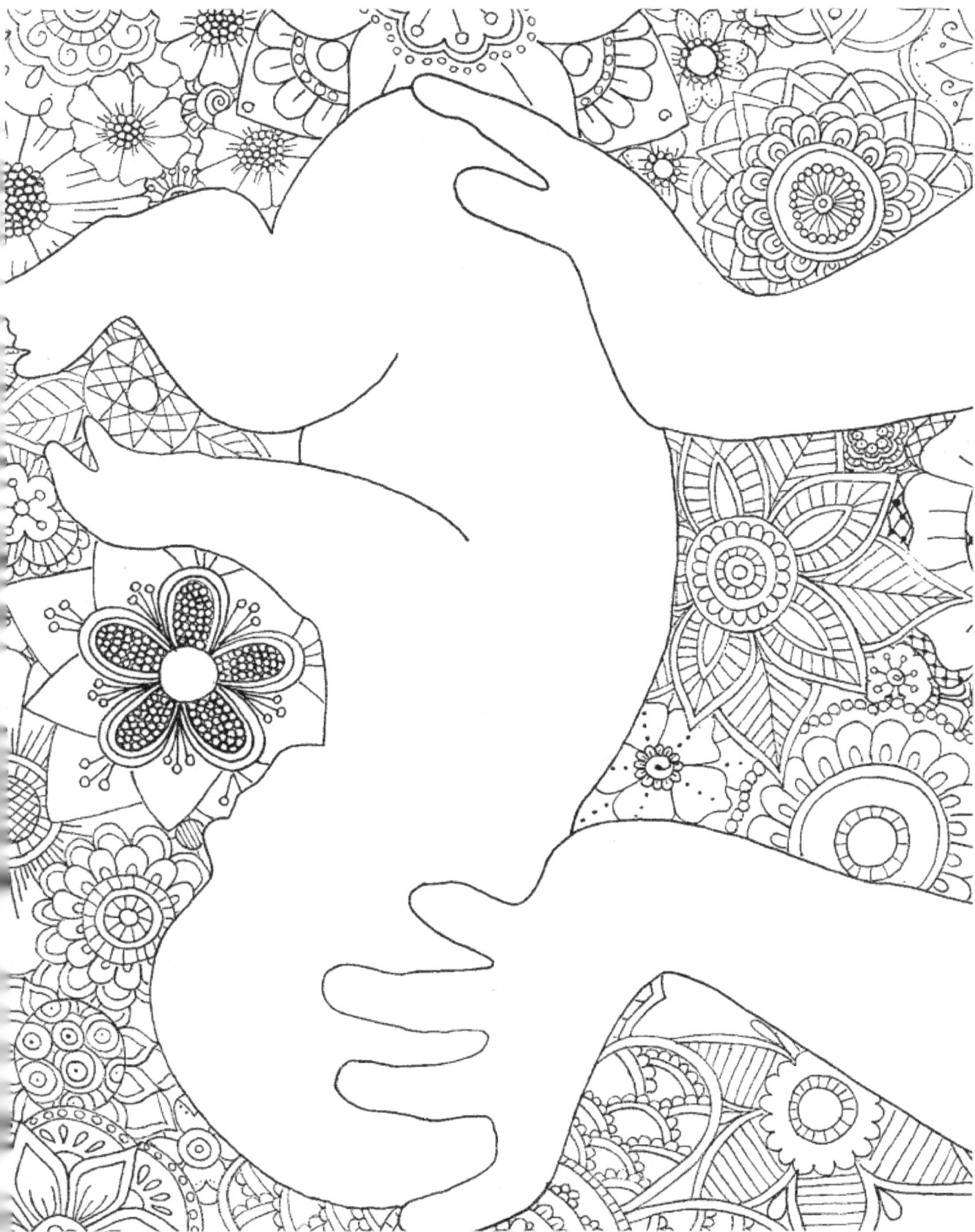

A mother is she who can take the place of all others but whose place no one else can take.

Gaspard Mermillod

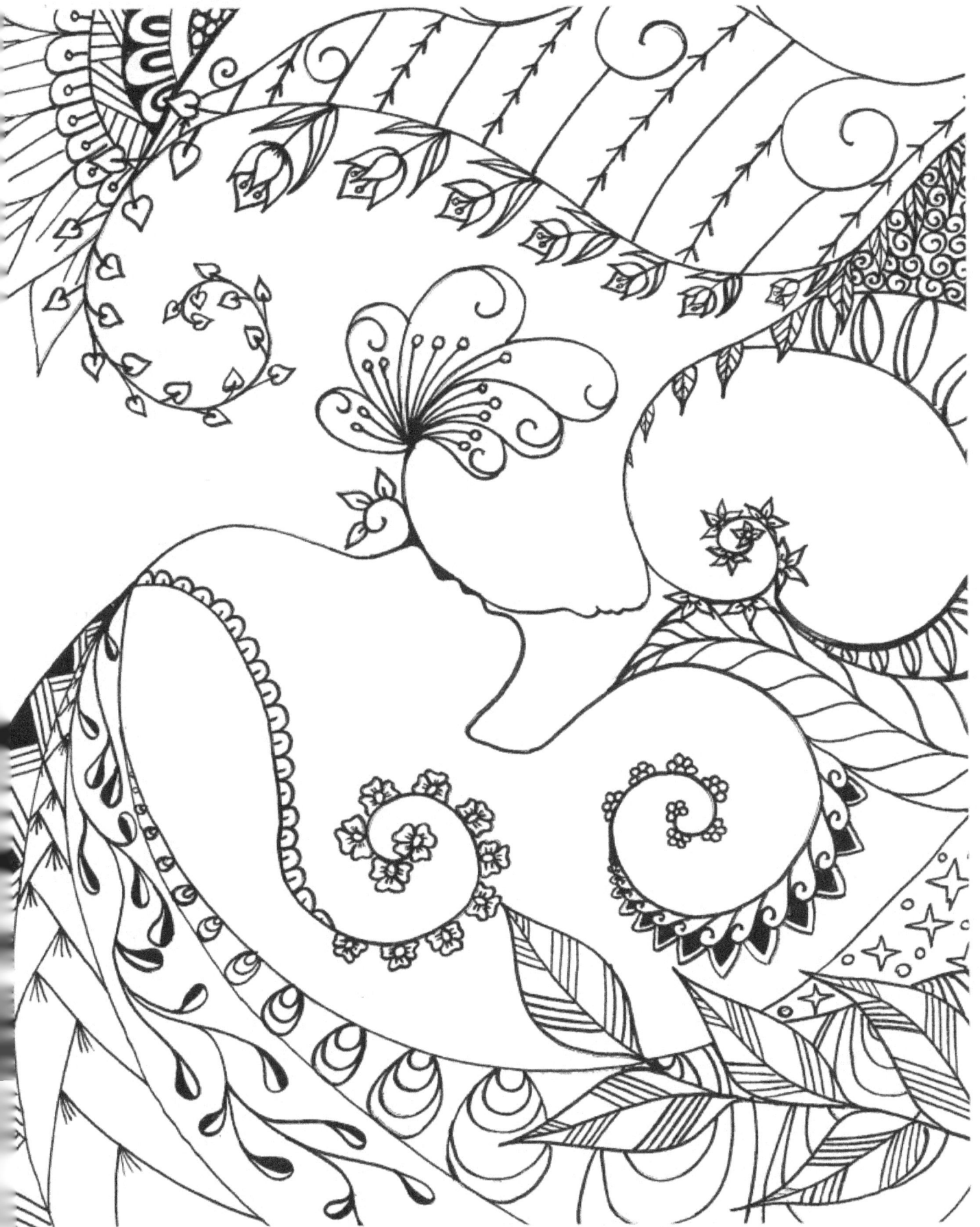

Motherhood is a choice you make every day, to put someone else's happiness and well-being ahead of your own, to teach the hard lessons, to do the right thing even when you're not sure what the right thing is... and to forgive yourself, over and over again, for doing everything wrong.

Donna Ball

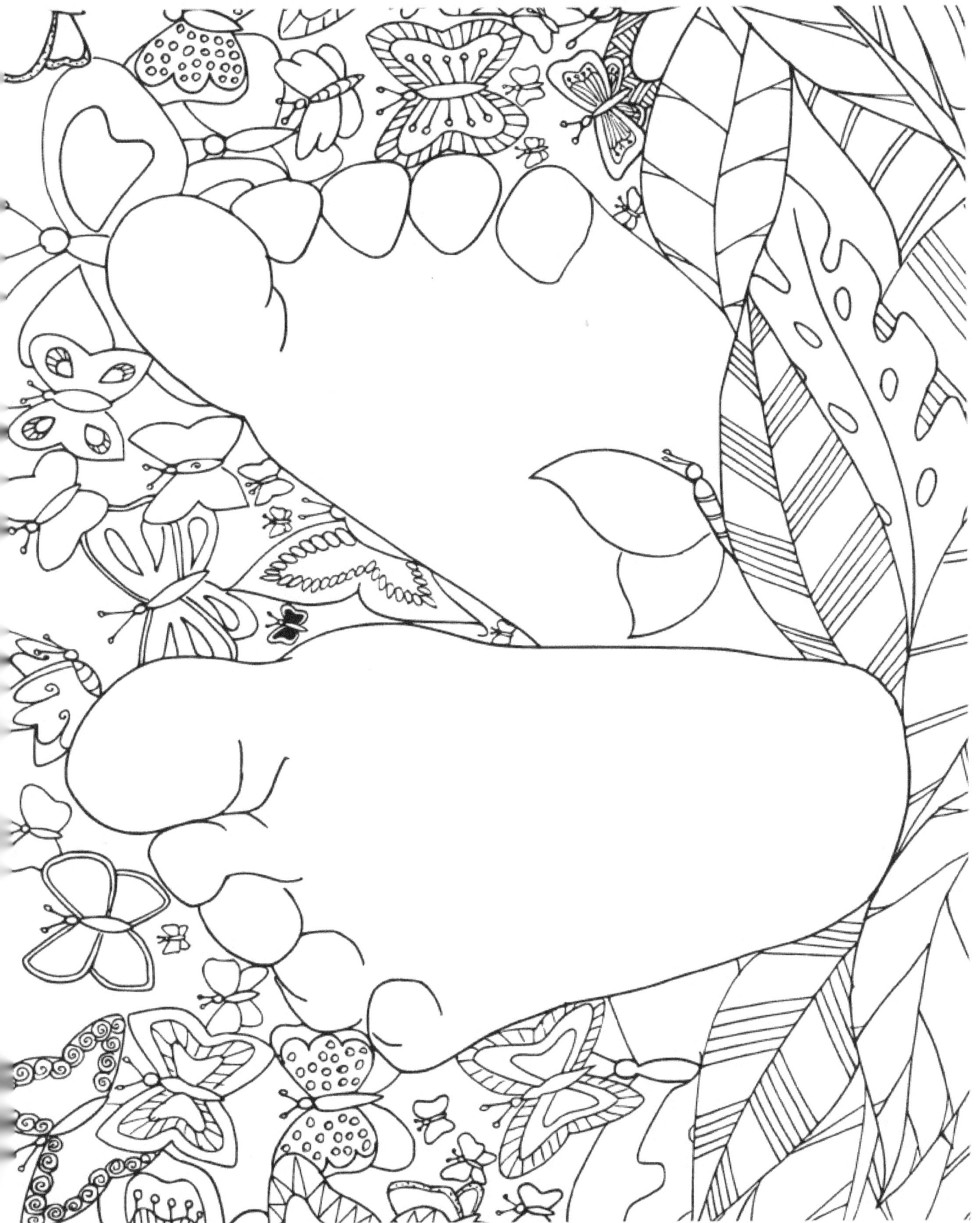

Mother's love is peace. It need not be acquired, it need not be deserved.

Erich Fromm

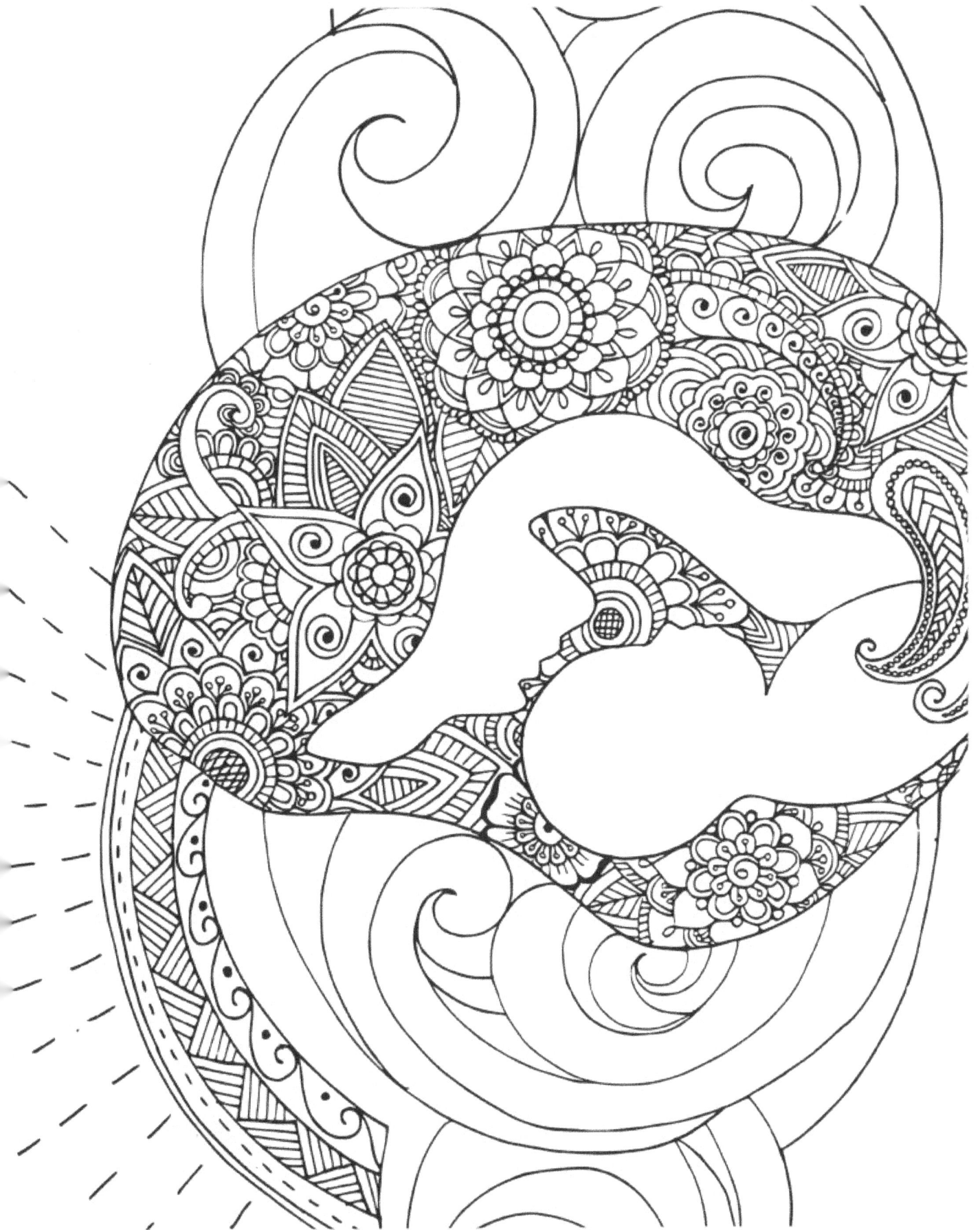

A mother is the truest friend we have, when trials heavy and sudden fall upon us; when adversity takes the place of prosperity; when friends desert us; when trouble thickens around us, still will she cling to us, and endeavor by her kind precepts and counsels to dissipate the clouds of darkness, and cause peace to return to our hearts.

Washington Irving

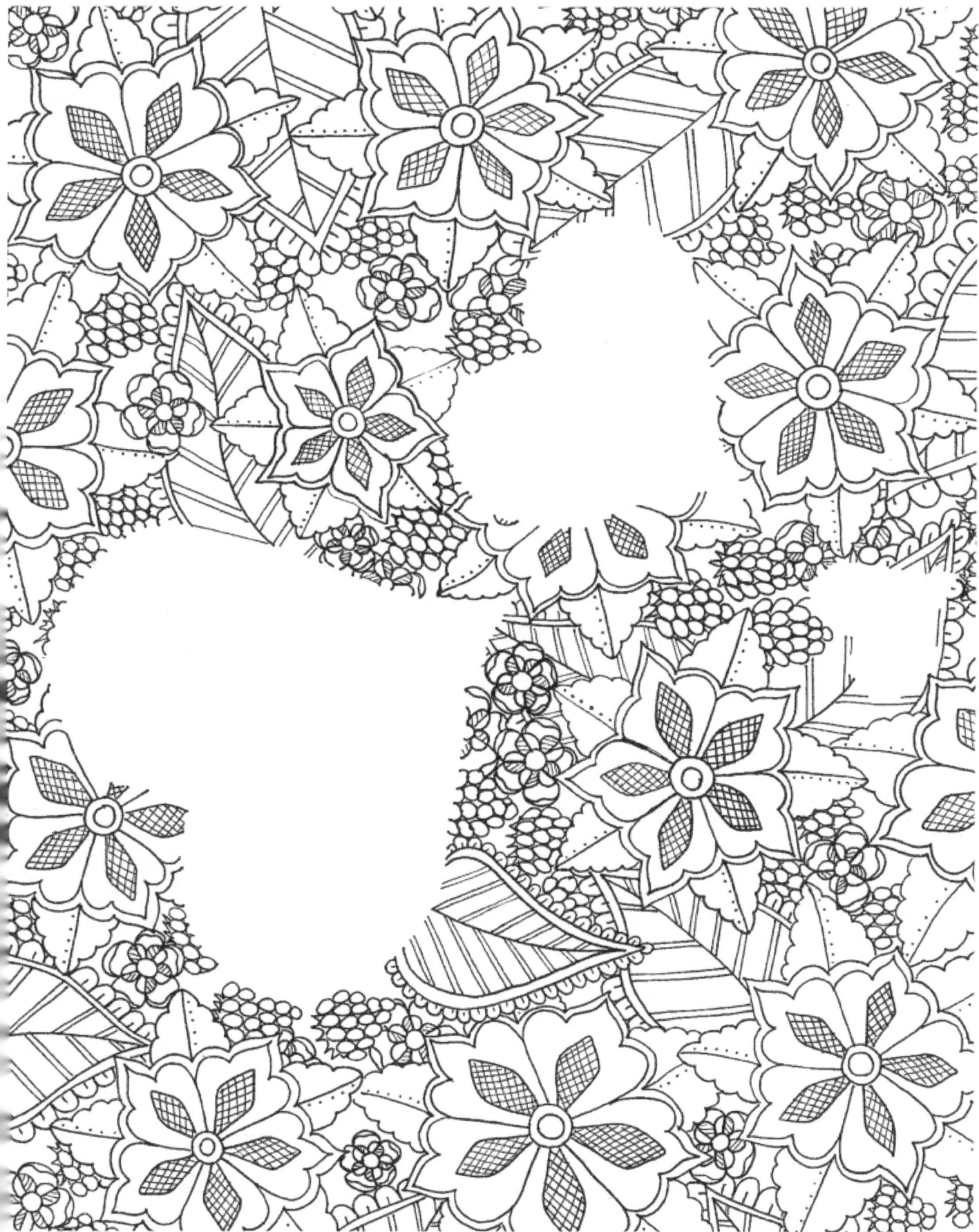

A newborn baby has only three demands. They are warmth in the arms of its mother, food from her breasts, and security in the knowledge of her presence. Breastfeeding satisfies all three.

Grantly Dick-Read

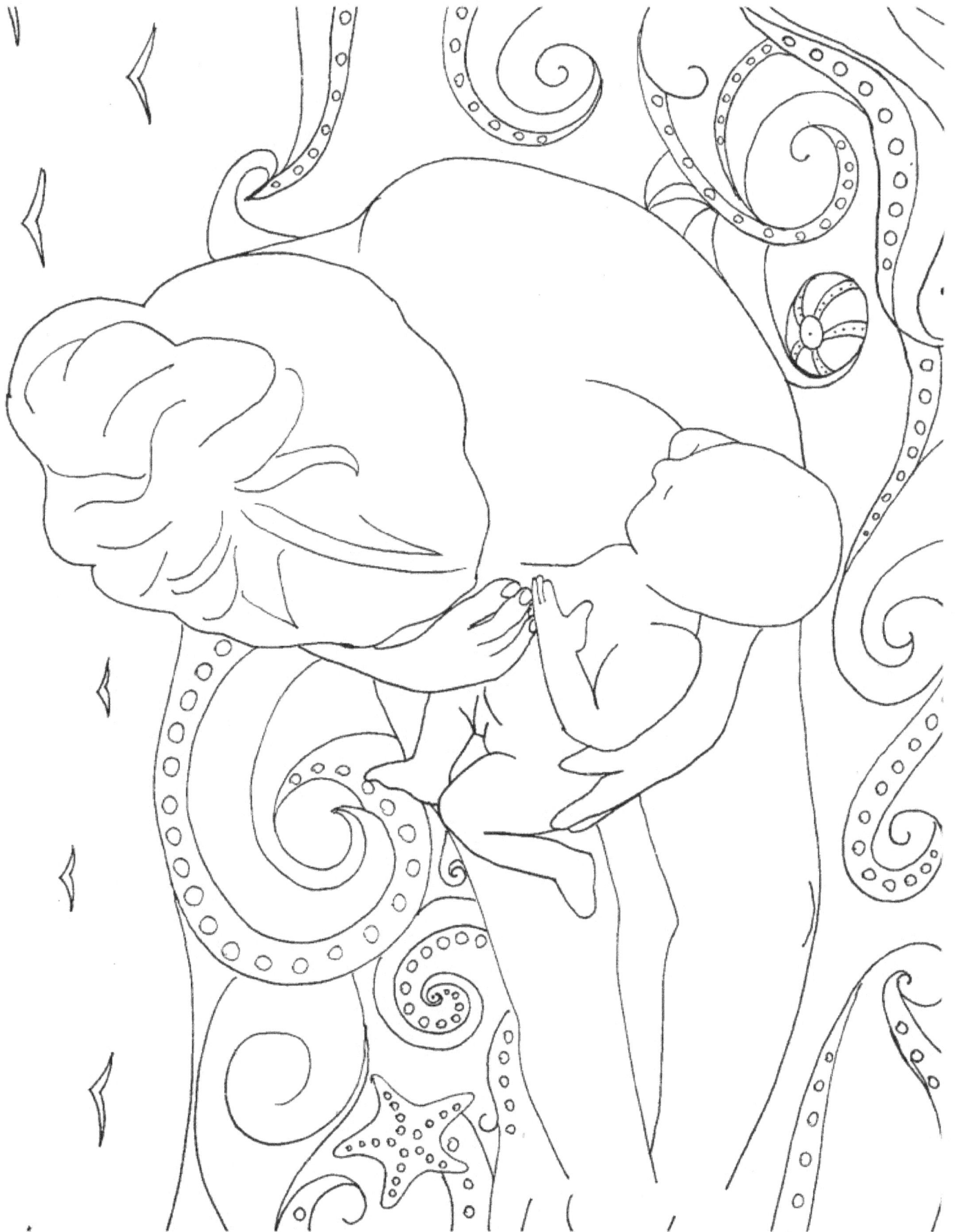

There is such a special sweetness in being able to participate in creation.

~Pamela S. Nadav

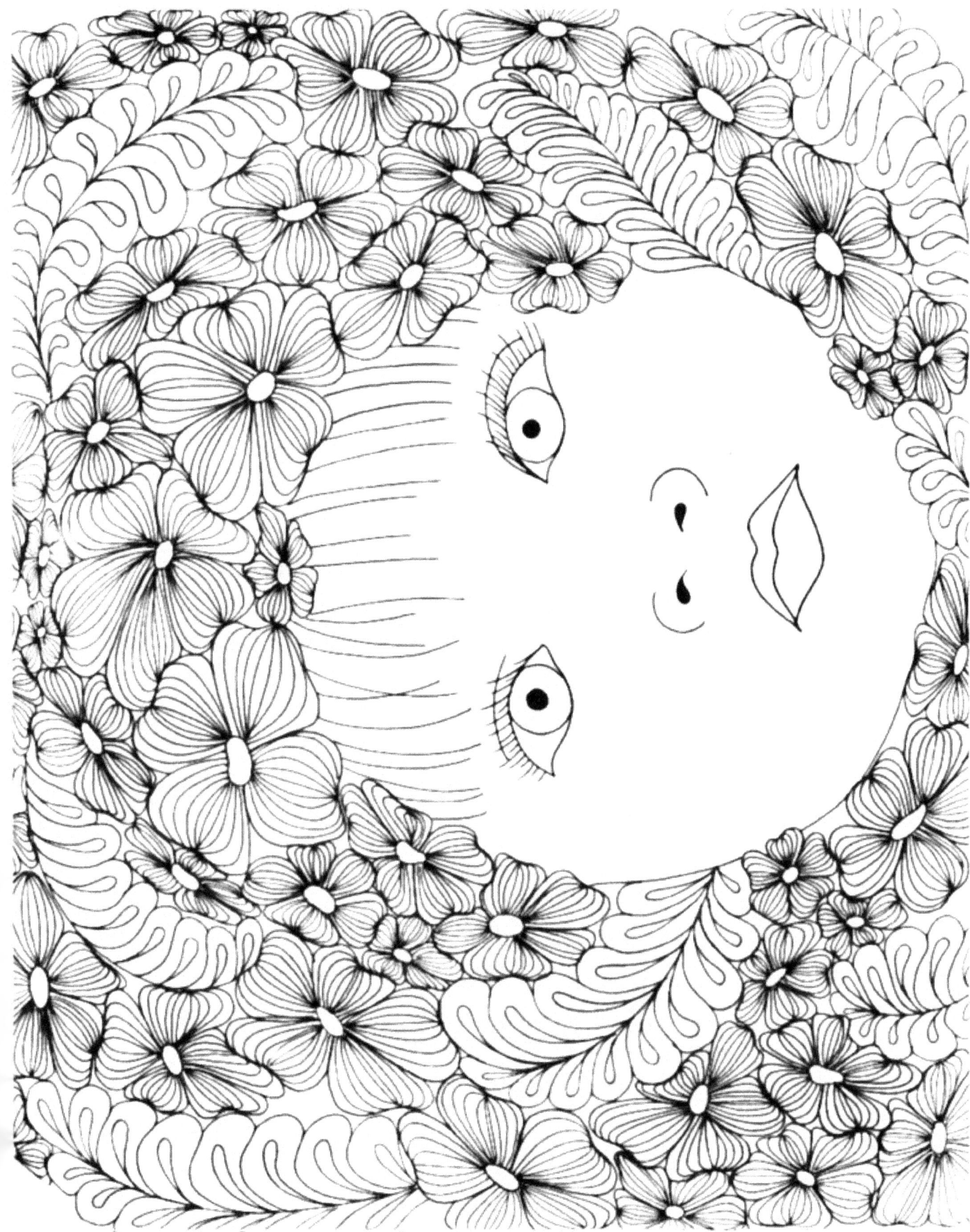

The natural power of breastfeeding is one of the greatest wonders of the world. It is about real love. It is about caring and celebrating the wondrous joy of nurturing a new life. It is about enjoying being a woman.

Anwar Fazal

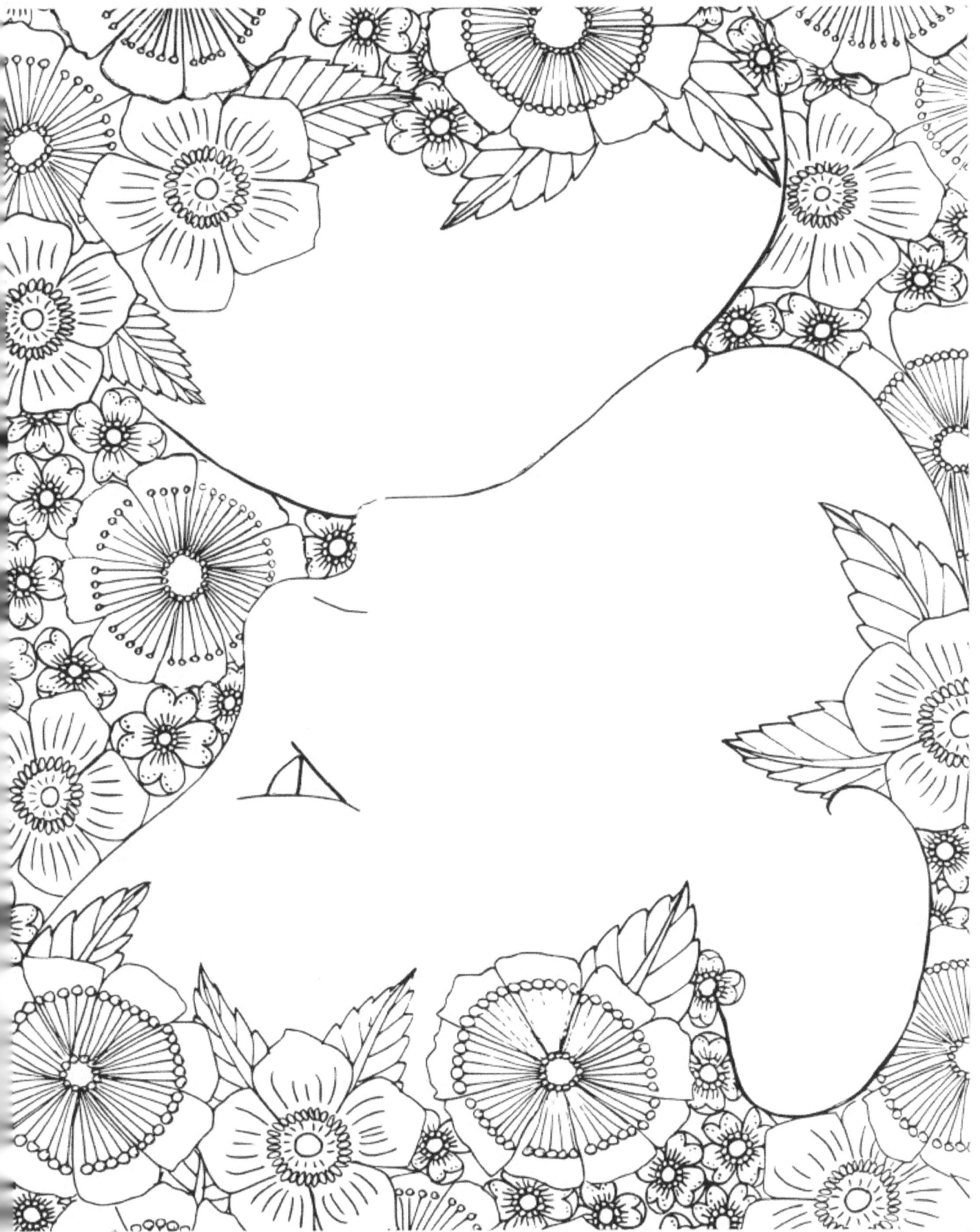

When the first baby laughed for the first time, the laugh broke into a thousand pieces and they all went skipping about, and that was the beginning of fairies. And now when every new baby is born it's first laugh becomes a fairy.

James Matthew Barrie

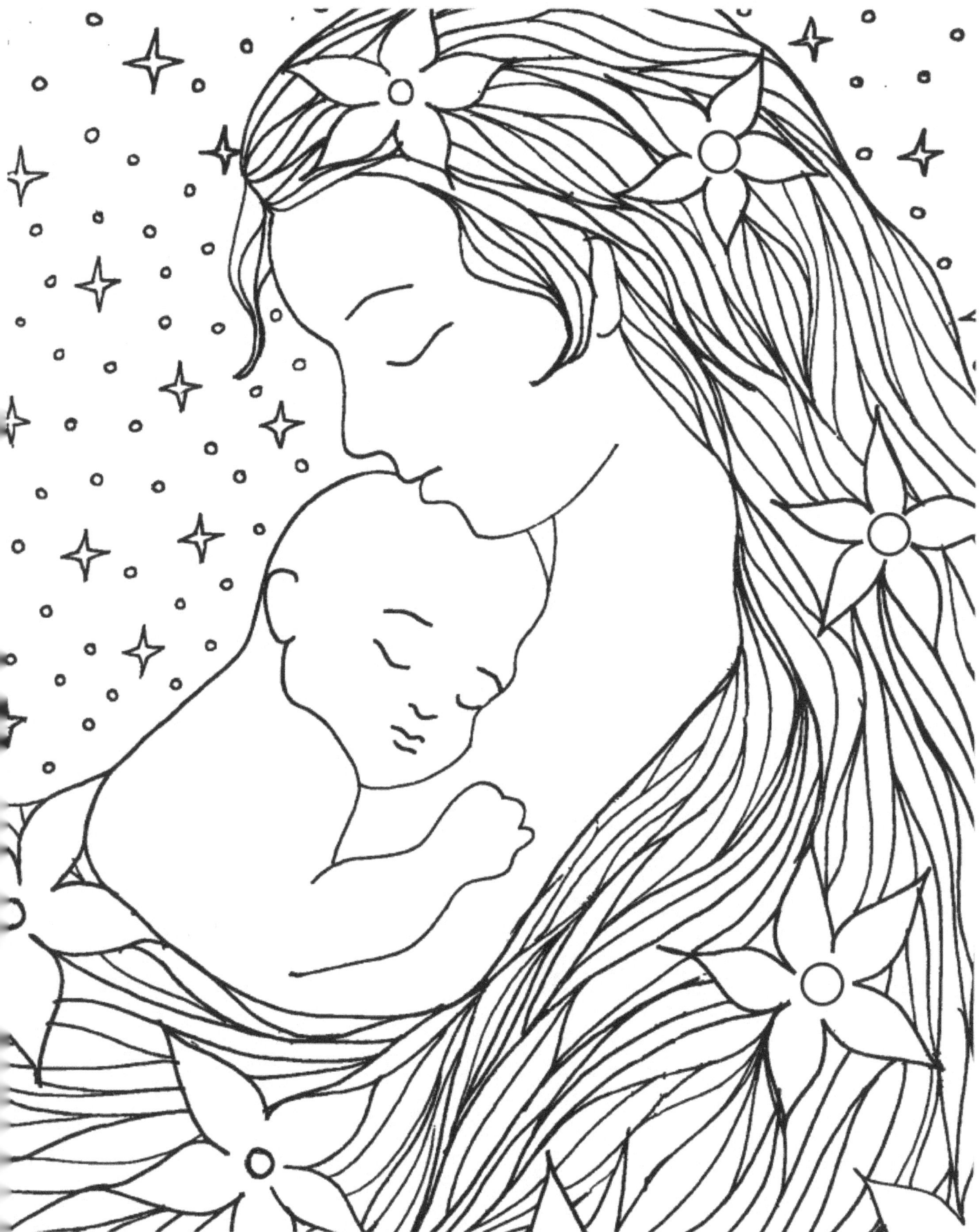

Breastfeeding is an unsentimental metaphor for how love works, in a way. You don't decide how much and how deeply to love - you respond to the beloved, and give with joy exactly as much as they want.

Marni Jackson

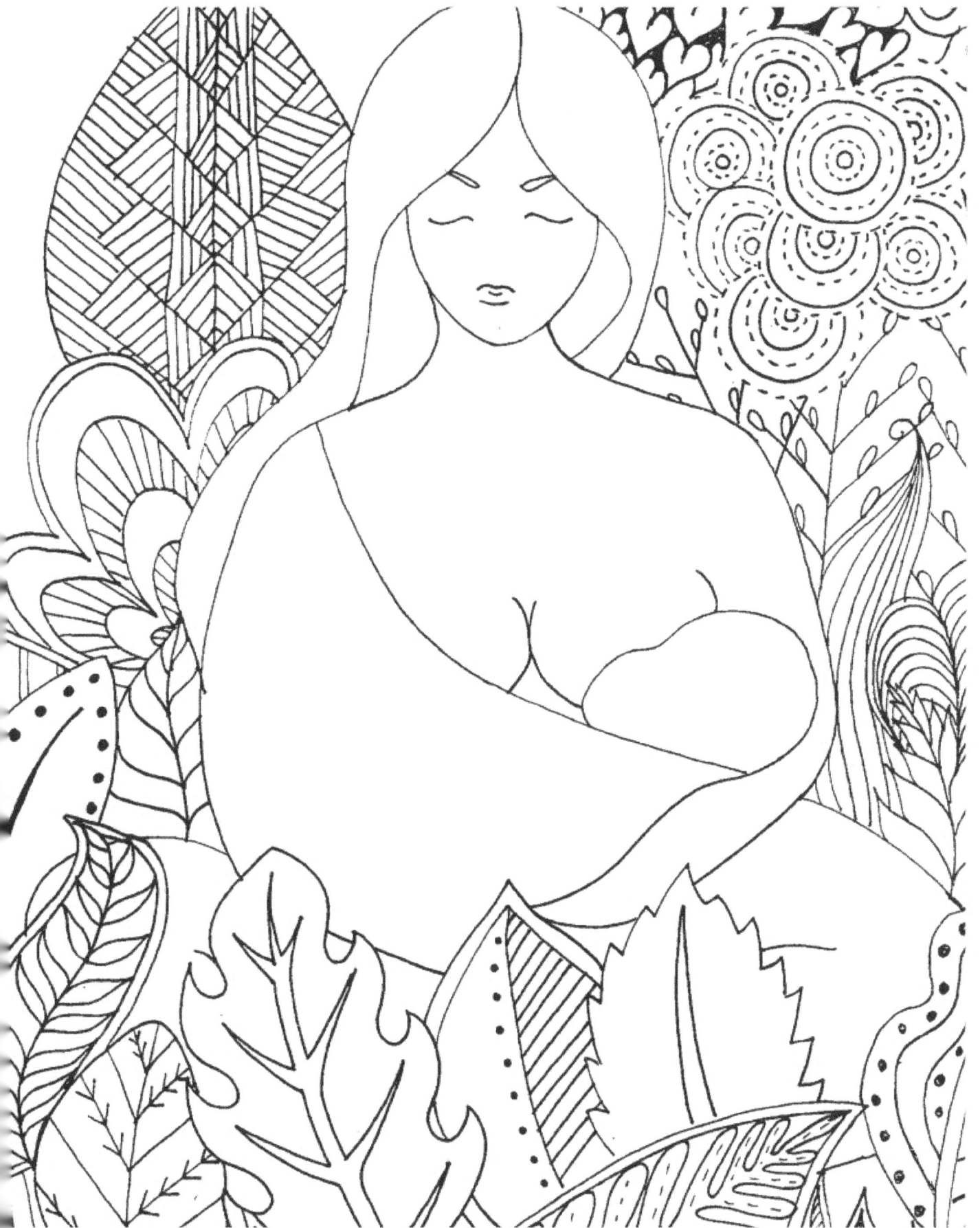

Mother is the name for God in the lips and hearts of little children.

William Makepeace Thackeray

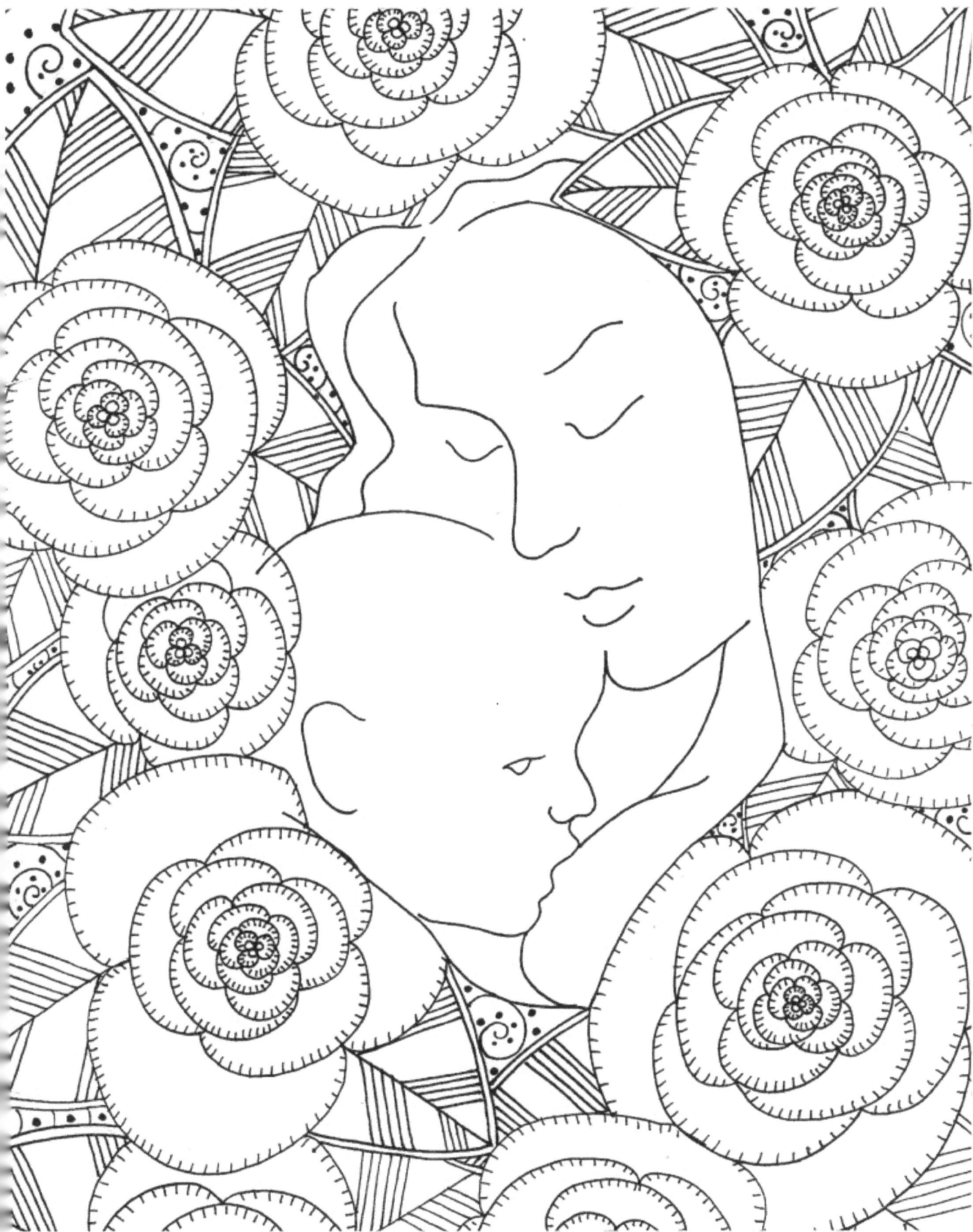

Life began with waking up and loving my mother's face.

George Eliot

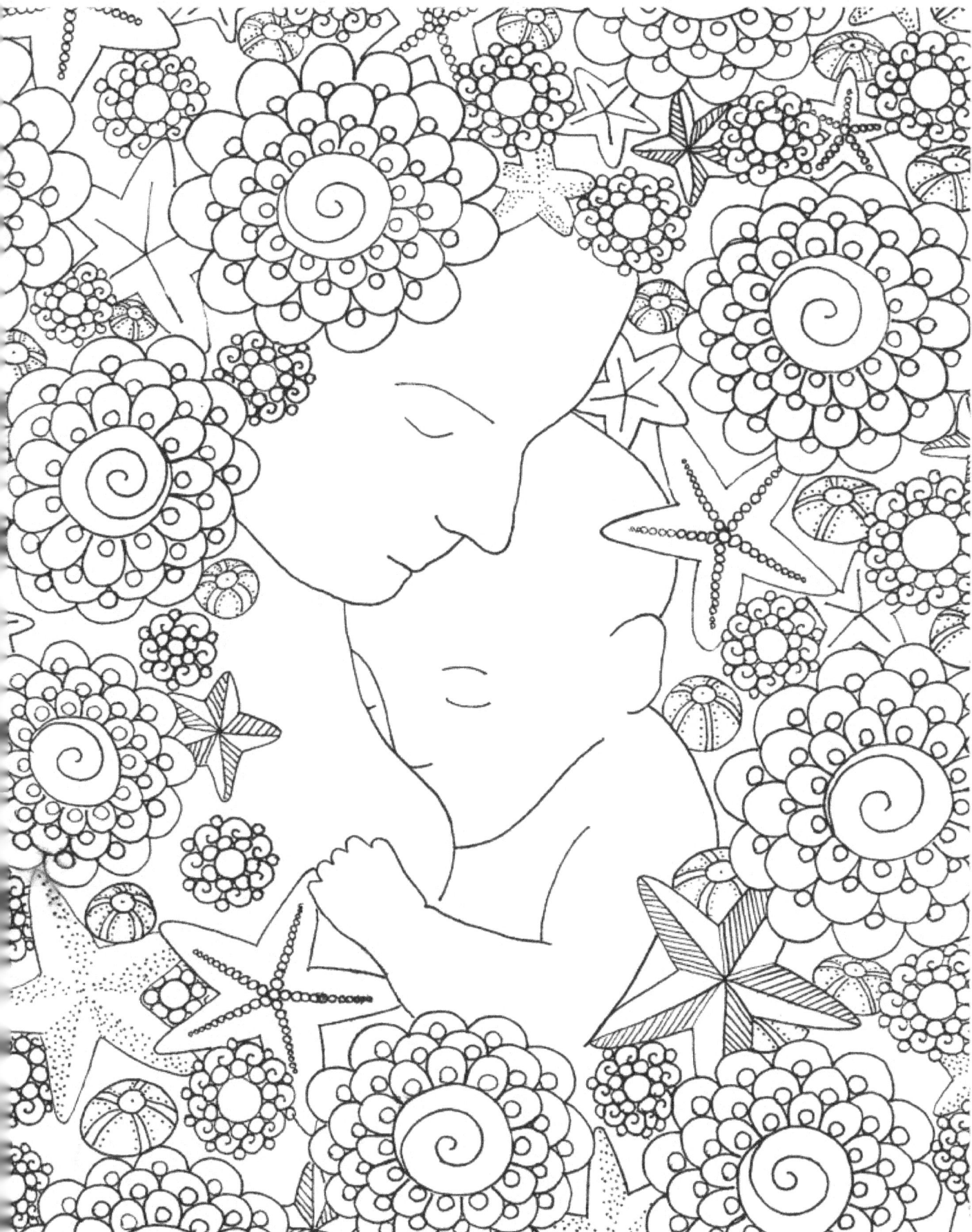

Mama was my greatest teacher, a teacher of compassion, love and
fearlessness. If love is sweet as a flower,
then my mother is that sweet flower of love.

Stevie Wonder

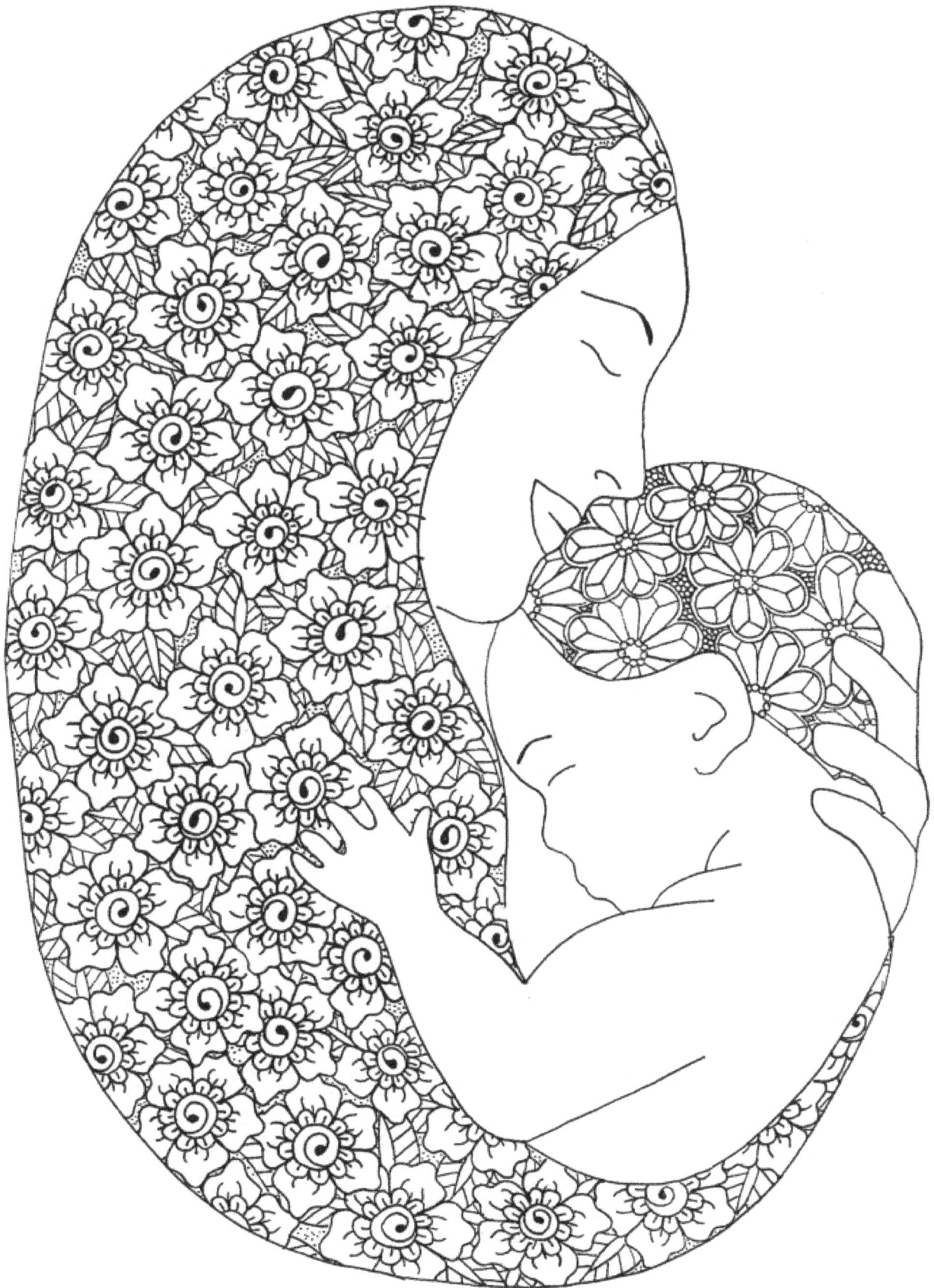

Babies are the buds of imagination that are ready to bloom with lights of love and affection.

Debasish Mridha

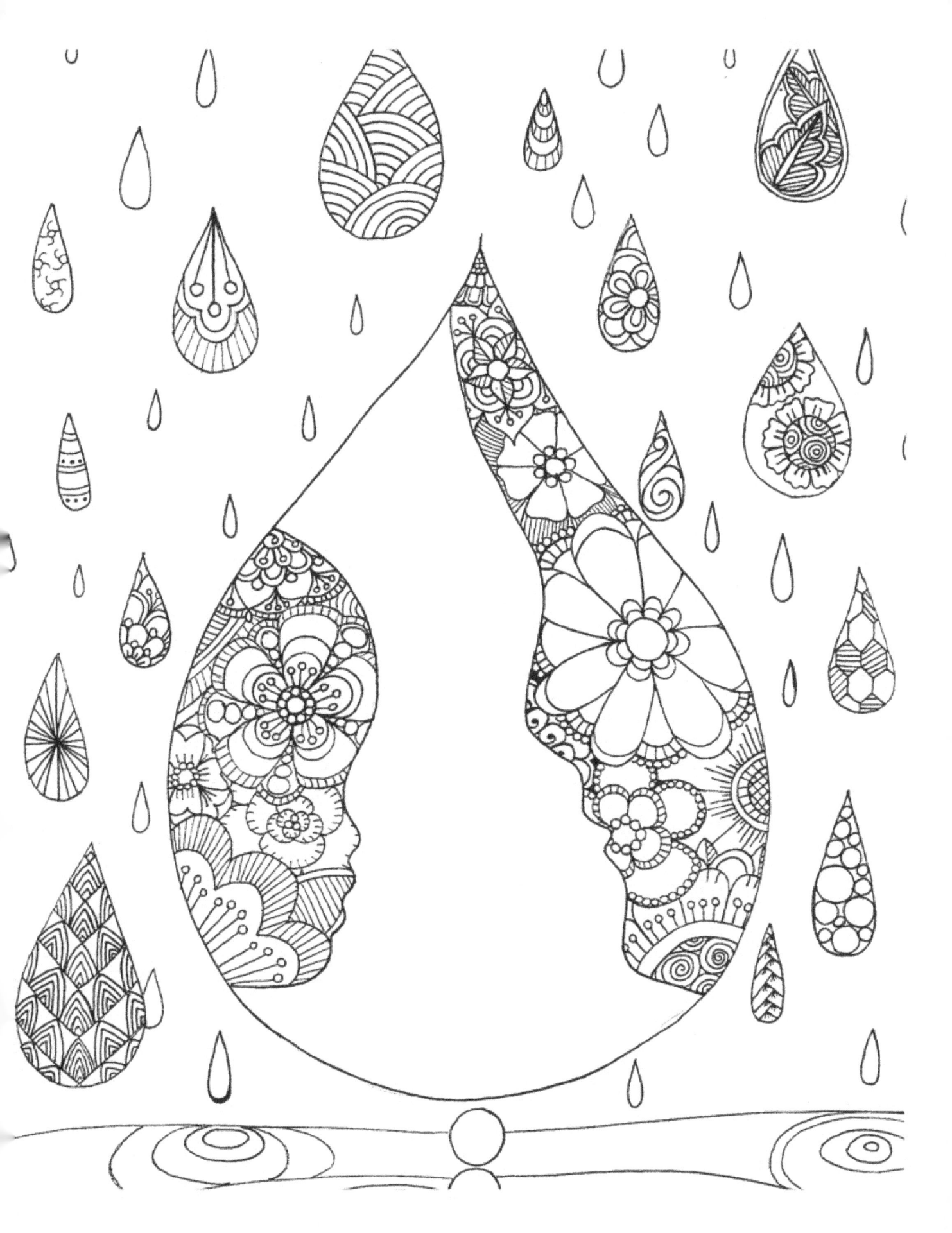

A little child born yesterday

A thing on mother's milk and kisses fed.

Homer

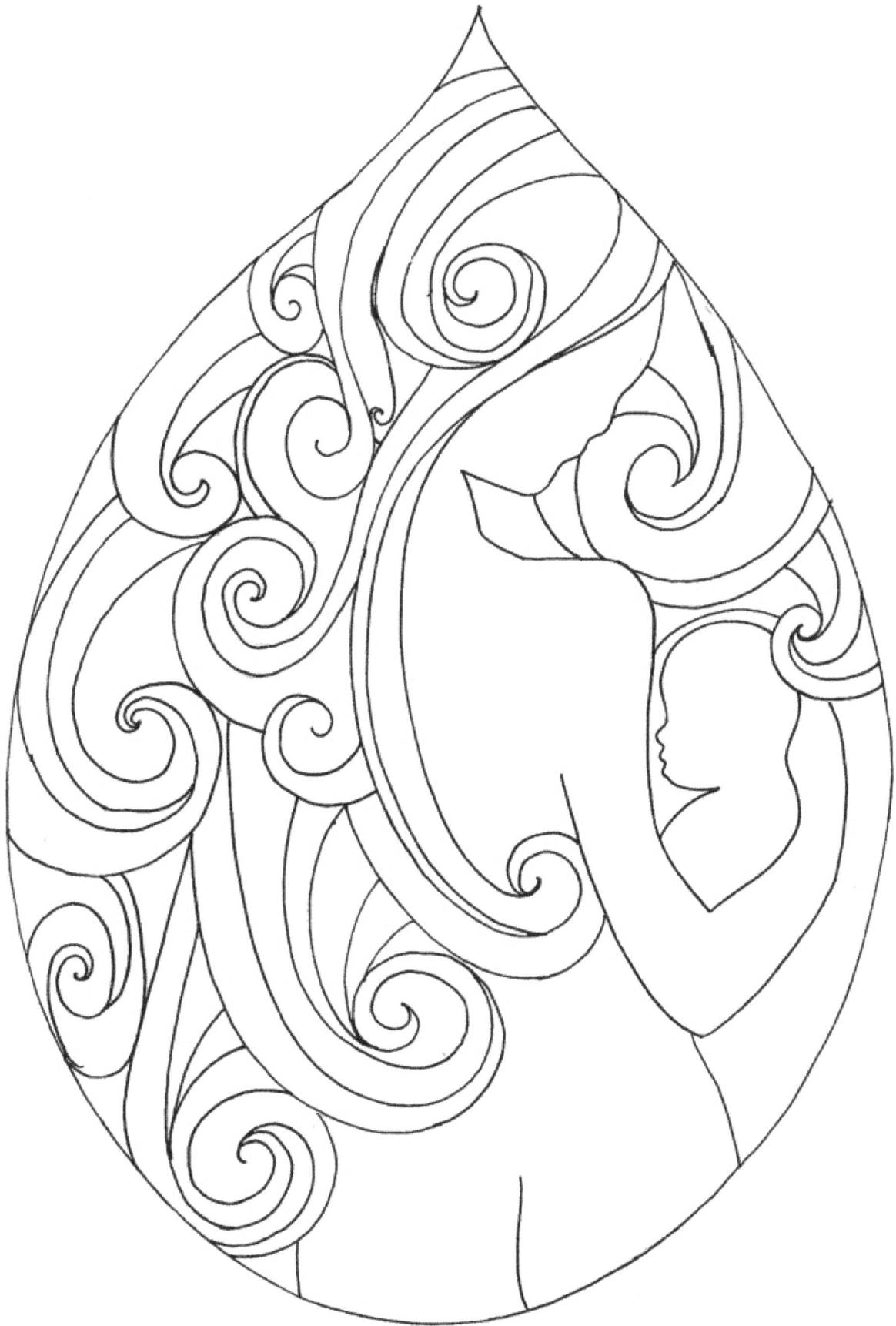

A new baby is like the beginning of all things wonder, hope,
a dream of possibilities.

Eda J. Le Shan

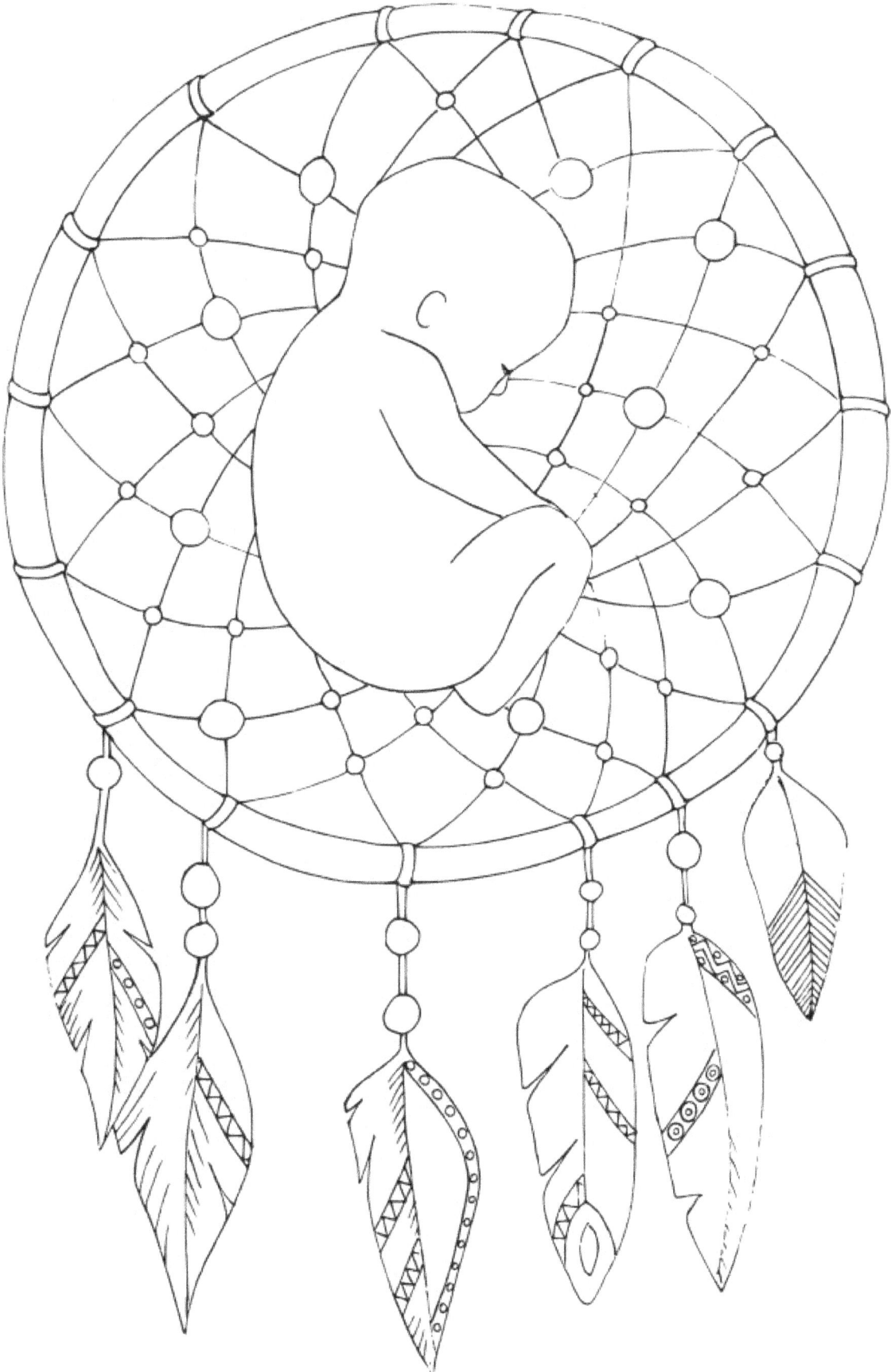

Fathering is the most masculine thing a man can do

Frank Pittman

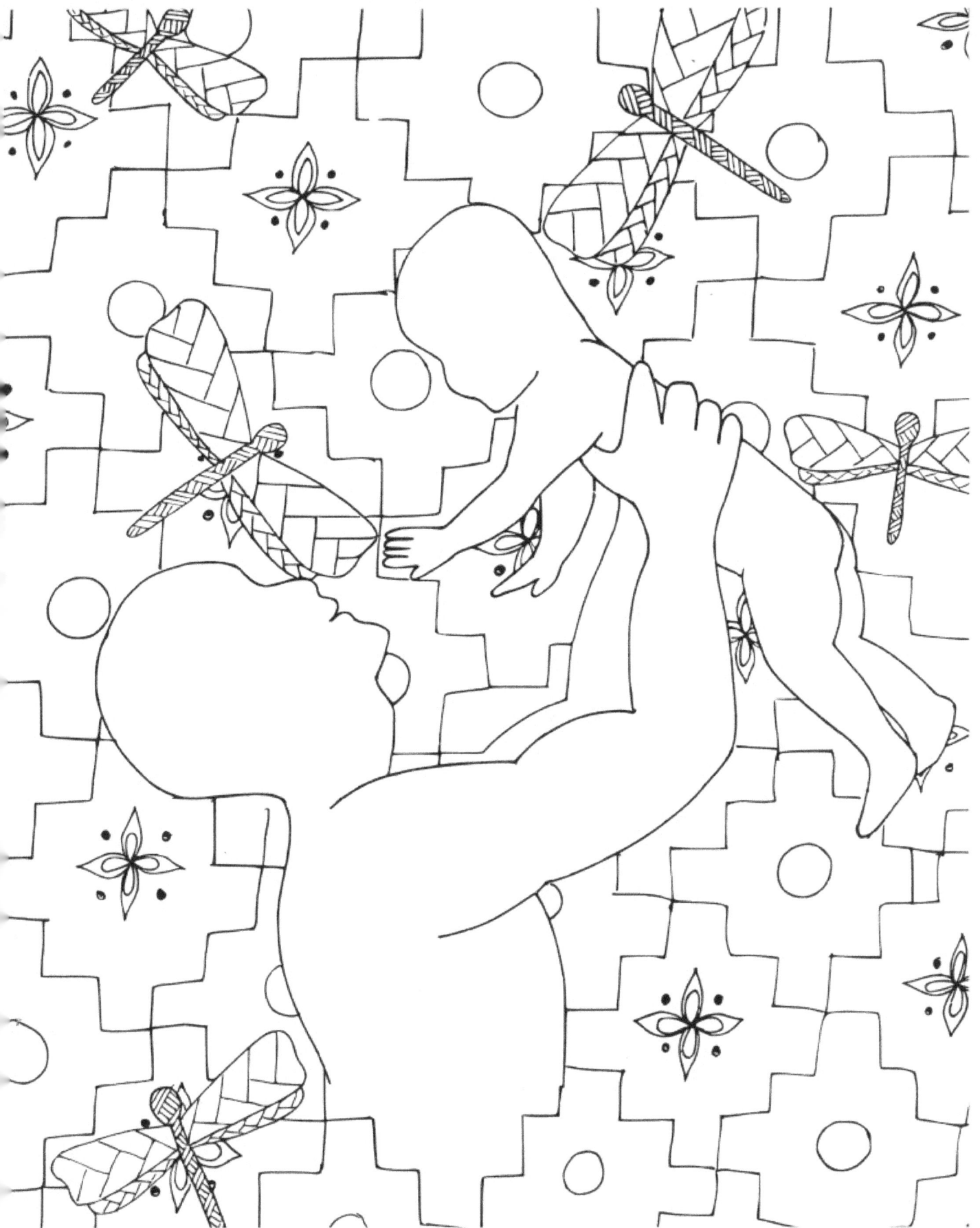

A good father is one of the most unsung, unpraised, unnoticed, and yet one of the most valuable assets in our society.

Billy Graham

ABOUT THE AUTHOR

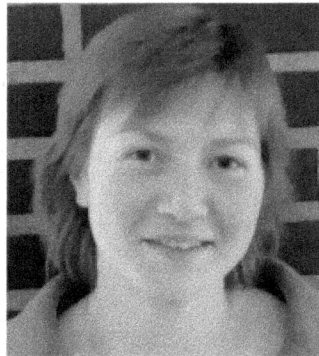

Mrs. Jemmais Keval-Baxter resides in Valdivia Chile with her family. She is a Professional Certified Prenatal, Labour and Postpartum Doula, Doula facilitator, EFT practitioner, writer, illustrator and Ho'oponopono coach. For more information about her books, services and workshops please consult her website at **www.hooponoponodoula.com** *and* **www.doulavaldivia.com**

www.ingramcontent.com/pod-product-compliance
Lightning Source LLC
Chambersburg PA
CBHW080021280326
41934CB00015B/3429